PREFACE

This text is designed for, and dedicated to, undergraduate students in nursing who are required to take a course in introduction to research. It is to be noted that the text is written for persons who are expecting to assume only one research role: utilizer of research findings in practice. The intent is to provide information about the logic of scientific inquiry generally, and the steps in the research process specifically, so that practicing nurses may learn to evaluate the technical soundness of research findings. Students are expected to become *critical* consumers of research results and are also encouraged to believe in the importance of theory and research as necessary bases for advanced nursing practice.

This is not a text for graduate students who are expected to be able to write proposals and to do research, except as they may wish to use it as a stepping stone to the more comprehensive texts. It is for undergraduates who must learn enough of the language and process of research to understand whether the investigator's conclusions are based in good design and therefore may be incorporated into practice activities.

Most professional nurses have neither the wish nor the skill to design and carry out research, and it is not the activity that earns the greatest rewards in clinical settings. The fact remains that *all* professional nurses must learn to read research studies in a critical manner, with a view to incorporating the findings into practice, if it is appropriate to do so. They must be able to identify errors in design or interpretation which will lead to the decision not to use the findings, if that is the decision which should be made.

The *science* of nursing advances only as *practice* is based in theory and research. The new knowledge obtained with such creativity and skill by the researcher is useful only if it is used by the clinicians. If the clinicians are not aware of the results because they do not read research journals, or if they do not understand the relationship of theory and research to nursing practice, the new knowledge simply exists. It is not tested in practice, and it does not advance either the science or the practice of nursing.

Investigators and clinicians on the whole have different and equally important skills, and they need each other. The practice of a professional nurse who cannot read research reports because she does not understand the language of research does not grow and is not corrected. Equally, the activities of an investigator are hampered if the study findings are not tested in other than experimental settings. The science also does not grow if it is not corrected by practice.

In the practice professions there is no need for every practitioner to be a research scientist. However, every practitioner must understand enough of the concepts of science and of practice that professional decisions are based in theory and research.

Nursing students are exposed to the concepts of practice throughout the educational experience. It is the intent in this text to provide them with enough information in a usable form to encourage some understanding of the concepts of scientific inquiry.

This understanding is more than, and is not dependent on, understanding statistics, although undergraduate students will find that they know more than they think they do about how to deal with the numerical findings presented by investigators. They have had arithmetic and a little algebra, they are familiar with the decimal system and the concept of positive and negative numbers, and they know that numbers increase and decrease in magnitude. They can understand many of the tabular presentations in the research reports with just this much background. Also, it is now the trend in nursing education to require students to take an introductory course in statistics at the undergraduate level, so they learn to calculate averages and consider the range of the scores.

Since it is the responsibility of the investigator to interpret the numbers, the discussion section of a research report ties the numerical findings to the concepts of the study in such a way that much nursing research can be read and understood without knowing a great deal about statistical analysis. For this book, the application of statistical tests to the values of the variables is simply presented as the second, and less important, analytic activity. No effort is made to address the statistical arithmetic. Students are advised to examine tables to get what information they can from them; at this level, they must depend on editors not to publish the studies in which the statistics are not appropriate to the data set.

Chapters 1 and 2 of the text contain an overview of the research process, in which the importance of research to a profession is presented, and the steps of the research process are presented in a logical chronology and defined. The rest of the chapters elaborate on the definitions, and discuss each of the steps in the process in the detail appropriate to an introductory text, up to the final chapter. Chapter 12 suggests the questions the reader should ask about the research report, and indicates what the answers must be in a technically sound design. The appendix provides an example of a critical review, using the questions developed in Chapter 12.

PRIMER

of
NURSING
RESEARCH

MARY REARDON CASTLES, R.N., Ph.D.

Professor and Director of Research,
School of Nursing,
University of Missouri—St. Louis

1987

W. B. SAUNDERS COMPANY

Philadelphia, London, Toronto, Mexico City,
Rio de Janeiro, Sydney, Tokyo, Hong Kong

W. B. Saunders Company: West Washington Square
                           Philadelphia, PA   19105

Library of Congress Cataloging-in-Publication Data

Castles, Mary Reardon.

Primer of nursing research.

Includes index.

1. Nursing—Research—Methodology.   I. Title. [DNLM:
1. Nursing.   2. Research—methods.   WY 20.6 C353p]

RT81.5.C37 1987   610.73′072   86–10160

ISBN 0–7216–1713–1

Editor: Dudley Kay

Developmental Editor: Alan Sorkowitz

Production Manager: Frank Polizzano

Manuscript Editor: Barbara Hodgson

Illustrator: Joan Sinclair

Primer of Nursing Research   ISBN   0–7216–1713–1

Last digit is the print number: 9   8   7   6   5   4   3   2

Each chapter contains chapter objectives, chapter summaries, and study activities specific to the chapter content. The study activities are related to the objectives: if the study tasks are accomplished, the chapter objectives will be met.

It is appropriate to note here that steps were taken to avoid language that could be interpreted as sexist, without using the double pronouns *he/she* and *his/her*. In a first draft, the choice of pronoun to refer to a nonsexist noun (e.g., the investigator, the student) was random. Reviewers found this disconcerting but applauded the effort toward a gender-free style. Therefore, a systematic random technique was used to assign pronouns to chapters, such that in the even-numbered chapters pronouns referring to gender-free nouns are masculine, and in the odd-numbered chapters they are feminine.

In summary, the book is for students and staff nurses who expect to remain in clinical nursing, who do not expect to design research studies, and who will make practice decisions based on the research findings of others.

MARY REARDON CASTLES

CONTENTS

11
ETHICAL CONSIDERATIONS

12
QUESTIONS FOR CRITICAL REVIEW

PRIMER
of
NURSING
RESEARCH

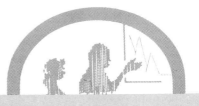

1

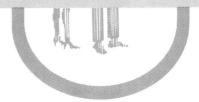

When you complete Chapter 1, you will be able to...

1. Defend the importance of research in nursing by
   a. Indicating how research can affect the credibility of nursing decisions.
   b. Indicating how research can affect nursing practice.

2. Identify the characteristics of a profession by
   a. Comparing nursing with law or medicine on each of the characteristics of a profession.

3. Differentiate research roles for practitioners by
   a. Providing examples of nurses observed in the various roles in an institutional setting.

4. Identify appropriate researcher-practitioner relationships by
   a. Describing researcher-practitioner relationships observed in an institutional setting.

ORIENTATION

THE IMPORTANCE OF RESEARCH IN NURSING

This book is designed to help students in undergraduate nursing programs come to grips with that mysterious activity known as "the research process." Nursing students who must know chemistry, biology, psychology, anthropology, and sociology, as well as nursing, in order to do their work, are perfectly capable of understanding the research process. It is not as mysterious as it seems and it can be a lot of fun. Even those students who do not intend to conduct research must learn enough about the process to be critical consumers of research findings, since nursing care plans should be changed on the basis of research findings, rather than on the basis of intuition or as a result of trial and error.

Nurses are trying to establish their credibility as professionals, and professionals have a research-based practice. Therefore, this section considers nursing as a profession.

Nursing is being moved toward professional status by a highly articulate portion of the membership. This movement is supported by the major nursing organizations. The question is no longer whether nursing is a profession, but how that status can be supported and defended to the membership and to the public.

There is not complete agreement as to the essential components of a profession that differentiate it from groups with less power and less prestige. Coe (1970) summarizes four characteristics that are *commonly* accepted and that can be considered for nursing. These are:

1. The expertise of the professional depends on an extensive body of theoretical knowledge.
2. The professional is committed to service.
3. A profession has a collegial organization rather than a bureaucratic one.
4. Professionals have both license and mandate.

The examination of nursing for these characteristics suggests that professionalism in nursing may still be, to some extent, potential rather than actual.

1. *The expertise of the professional depends on an extensive body of theoretical knowledge.* For nursing, as for medicine, this body of knowledge is not specific to the discipline. The theories of natural science support the activities of physicians, engineers, and, to some extent, nurses, although the paths from chemistry and biology to nursing frequently lead through medicine. The theories of social science support the activities of nurses and some physicians, lawyers, and theologians. However, that portion of the body of knowledge of nursing derived from these theories is specific to nursing only in the application of the theoretical information. Theories in nursing have recently been elaborated to the extent that nursing education and nursing practice can be based in many of them, although all of them require further testing to determine whether they should provide bases for education and practice.

2. *The professional is committed to service.* This commitment is central to the concept of professionalism; the professional is expected to place the needs of clients above personal preferences or needs. This expectation has always been common in nursing and is probably the only characteristic that is considered by the public, by health care system colleagues, and by all nurses to be a necessary component of nursing. Although there probably would not be agreement that the needs of clients *are* always placed first, all share the expectation that they should be.

3. *A profession has a collegial organization rather than a bureaucratic one.* This characteristic is no longer to be perceived in its pure form, even in the older professional groups. The bureaucracy of the church, of the courts, and of the hospitals affects the decisions of even the most collegial pastors, lawyers, and physicians. Nurses, who have always been employees, are perhaps more fortunate than their elder brothers in professionalism in that they have learned to serve two masters: the profession and the employing institution. Professional organizations themselves have become so formalized, so large and powerful, that they constitute a bureaucratic threat to collegial socialization and decision. Although there has been some movement into independent practice, most nurses are employed by an institution

or a group, and therefore are vulnerable to conflict between professional and bureaucratic values.

4. *Professionals have both license and mandate.* License confers the right to practice and to impart special knowledge; *mandate* refers to the right of the profession to declare the standards of practice. In nursing, three kinds of educational experience, only one of which is university-based, may lead to the license; the mandate is open to medical interference and employer constraints in most health care settings. There is, therefore, some question as to the quality of this characteristic in the profession of nursing.

Styles (1982) addresses the subject by differentiating the concepts of professionalism and professionhood. She defines professionalism as that which characterizes a profession but suggests that nurses focus on professionhood, the characteristics of the individuals who are members of a profession, since professionalism is achieved only through the professionhood of the members. She identifies a set of characteristics commonly ascribed to professions that are similar to Coe's summary: an extensive university education, a unique body of knowledge, a service orientation, a professional organization, and autonomy and self-regulation. Self-regulation is sometimes equated with the development and publication of a code of ethics, and nursing has taken this step. Autonomy, which may be the "key value" (p. 27) of a profession, is not so clearly in place.

Whether professionalism in nursing is potential or actual, the importance of research to nursing can be considered in terms of the status of the profession and the status of the practice. An occupation does not become a profession without research-based, advanced practice. Research that evaluates nursing practice, that identifies what nurses do, how they do it, and what happens to clients because it is done is a necessary precursor to the advancement of the practice.

Polit and Hungler (1983) suggest that the ultimate goal of any profession is to improve the practice of its members. Implicit in this is the identification and elaboration of a body of knowledge that is specific to nursing. This will occur through the continuing development of the explanatory and predictive principles of nursing theories; however, research that will simply organize some part of the aggregate of facts currently constituting the body of knowledge of nursing is also necessary.

Nursing has a long history, and many of the acts of nursing are based in traditions of care that have not been subjected to question until recently. Certainly, many of the acts of nursing are not well understood, even by those persons most involved in them. Understanding can come through research, which provides descriptions of and support for nursing activities. The evolution of a profession and the advancement of practice come primarily

as a result of knowledge developed and enlarged through research.

Nursing research that addresses clinical variables and is
carried out in clinical settings advances nursing practice, but
only if research findings are given intelligent use by practitioners.
The solution of nursing problems requires some understanding
of how they come about and how they persist. The techniques of
research offer a way of examining and understanding the operation of human affairs (Babbie, 1979), and therefore the operation
of the acts of nursing.

If nursing is to be a profession, and if the baccalaureate
degree is to be the entry credential, then an introduction to the
concepts and methods of research is required at the baccalaureate
level. In a practice discipline, research is necessary to build the
science that will direct the practice: the practitioners must be
able to understand the process in order to evaluate and use (or
not use) the findings.

RESEARCH ROLES FOR PRACTITIONERS

Despite a somewhat passionate literature identifying the need
for research in nursing, and despite the housing of professional
education in university settings, most nurses are not involved in
nursing research. In the usual nursing service setting, research is
not likely to be seen as a legitimate use of staff time by either of
the two most powerful persons in the professional life of staff
nurses: the nursing supervisor and the physician. Even in aca-
deme, the concept of "released time" to do research indicates
that it is not such an integral part of faculty professional life as
are students and committees. The research staff or the faculty
may be set aside in some, not always explicit way: patient care
needs and student learning needs are really what nurses in the
two settings are being paid to consider. There is indeed some
question whether it is appropriate for all practitioners to be
research oriented, but regardless of whether it is appropriate, in
nursing it is certainly not realistic.

Notter (1974) identified multiple research roles for nurses
and suggested that it is not necessary for all nurses to learn to
fill each and every one. The role of the principal investigator,
who designs studies and carries them out, is not for everyone,
and in the past, the nurse who developed the skill to do this was
usually required to give up clinical aspirations. The skills were
not to be found in most nursing curricula; some interdisciplinary
crossover was required. Today, when the doctorate in nursing
may be earned at 30 or more universities, clinical skill need not
be sacrificed to obtain research skill. However, not all nurses
wish to take the time or make the effort, and perhaps move away
from clinical expertise, to become principal investigators. Those

who have done so usually work in academic settings, although an increasing number are developing the role of the research nurse in clinical settings.

A second role in nursing research is to facilitate the research activities of a principal investigator. Nurses in the clinical setting who serve as data collectors and as subjects—and in so doing find out how a study is conducted—fulfill this role, as does a head nurse who allows the investigator on the unit and a director of nursing who authorizes the study. It is a role in which much may be learned, and because clinical investigators cannot function without such facilitation, it is vital to the research effort.

The third research role is one that every professional nurse must assume as a matter of course: the use of research results in nursing practice. Until professional nursing is based on an understanding and use of the empirical findings of nursing research, or on verified nursing theory, there can be little advanced practice. All professional nurses must, therefore, learn to be critical consumers of research results. They must be able to review the studies reported in the research journals as well as those reported in the clinical journals. It is necessary to be informed about the research process in order to understand research reports: this book provides that information.

THE INVESTIGATOR-PRACTITIONER RELATIONSHIP

A scientific practice base means that nursing practice is dictated by nursing theory or by empirical clinical research findings. It is necessary for nurses in active clinical practice to have input into the decisions which will determine the domain of that practice. The important task of generating research questions cannot be left to theorists, educators, or researchers, all of whom are firmly based in an academic rather than a clinical setting. This suggests the need for a certain kind of relationship between practitioners and researchers.

One of the possible research roles for nurses described earlier was that of participating in research conducted by others. The most important activity in that role is the definition of the clinical problems and the clinical variables, along with some ranking of their importance to practice by the clinician, for the investigator.

The practicing nurse knows which clinical questions should be answered; the researcher, given the information about the important clinical variables, can formulate research problems, write research questions or hypotheses to be tested, and develop the necessary designs. Practitioners identify the problems: practitioners use the findings. Between these two events, the researchers must first carry out technically sound studies to generate valid findings and then share the findings in a way that is useful to the practitioners. Generally, researchers have a bad habit—

they speak only with other researchers and not much with clinicians and nursing administrators.

Researchers assume that they need only report their findings, and that someone else is responsible for incorporating them into the health care system. Findings are either published in the research journals or reported at conferences to other researchers. Practitioners who might be interested in using the results do not subscribe to the research journals, nor do they attend the conferences. Therefore, findings are not translated into practice; this means that findings are not evaluated by the clinicians, and investigators never really know if their work has added to nursing knowledge. Practitioners remain skeptical of the importance of research in nursing, and a corrective process important in both research and practice is not carried out.

The primary relationship between investigator and practitioner should be one of information exchange and free use of each other's skills. The working relationship should be such that clinical nurses identify clinical problems and nurse investigators design studies to address these problems. Useful findings may be generated, which are returned to the clinical nurses. Critical review of the findings by that group, with an eye to use, can correct both the nursing care plan and the research design. This book provides enough information about the concepts and the process of research design that such critical review to precede use can be done by practicing nurses. Students will learn some of the vocabulary of a new language.

References

Babbie, E.R. The Practice of Social Research. 2d ed. Belmont, Calif.: Wadsworth, 1979.

Coe, R. Sociology of Medicine. New York: McGraw-Hill, 1970.

Notter, L.E. Essentials of Nursing Research. New York: Springer, 1974.

Polit, D., and B. Hungler. Nursing Research : Principles and Methods. 2d ed. Philadelphia: J.B. Lippincott, 1983.

Styles, M. On Nursing: Toward a New Management. St. Louis: C.V. Mosby, 1982.

Study Activities

1. Compare nursing with one of the accepted professional groups (e.g., medicine, law, theology) on the accepted characteristics of a profession.

2. Styles has written that autonomy is a *key value* for a profession. Identify nursing acts that may be considered autonomous.

3. Choose one of the three research roles identified and indicate whether that role could be carried out in your clinical setting. If it could be, describe how. If it could not be, identify the characteristics of the setting that preclude research roles for nurses.

4. Identify the relationship that exists between researchers and practitioners in your setting. Indicate how it might be changed in the direction of the cooperative interaction described in the text.

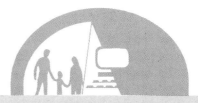

2

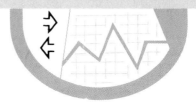

When you complete Chapter 2 you will be able to...

1. Describe nursing as a science by
   a. Discriminating among the various meanings of the word science.
   b. Indicating how each of the meanings may apply to nursing.

2. Describe the logical progression toward a research design by
   a. Discriminating among the conceptual, empirical, and interpretive phases of the process.
   b. Listing and defining the steps of the research process that are likely to occur in each phase.

THE RESEARCH PROCESS

APPROACHES TO SCIENTIFIC INQUIRY

One of the difficulties in understanding and using a new language is that some words have more than one meaning. The word science has several separate, distinct, but related, meanings. Four of these are:

1. a branch of systematized knowledge, considered as a distinct field of investigation or an object of study.

2. the observation and classification of facts leading to the establishment of testable general laws.

3. accumulated and accepted knowledge, classified and made available.

4. a system purporting to be based on scientific principles, reconciling practical ends with scientific laws.

The various nursing theories provide systematized knowledge in a distinct field (definition 1) as well as scientific principles than can be taken to the practice setting to see if they work (definition 4). Nursing acts, presently based in common sense, intuition, and what has been found to be effective, constitute an area of study in which general laws of nursing are established and tested (definition 2); nursing also requires classification (definition 3). A reference to nursing science, therefore, may be a reference to the theories, the derived laws, the frameworks that relate the laws to the theories and to the clinical setting, the effort to identify and classify nursing acts (e.g., the work with nursing diagnosis), or the effort to generate general laws from the aggregate of facts that constitute a major portion of the body of knowledge of nursing.

Nursing is a developing science, and in this book, it is considered to be a social science. The research designs and data-collection instruments to be discussed are taken from the social science disciplines. In the natural sciences, the "experiment" is the rule, and nothing else is likely to be considered research. Researchers in nursing do not always have the luxury of working only under well-controlled conditions in laboratories, and designs that allow investigators to do research in clinical and other real-life settings are required. Laboratory-based findings do not always transfer to the untidy world, and a nursing science that only works under laboratory conditions is not a useful science for practitioners. This is not to say that laboratory-based research findings are not an important part of the science and the practice of nursing, merely to suggest that the laboratory is not the only setting that is proper for nursing research.

Nursing is considered a social science for two reasons: the nursing act is an interaction between people, not between cells or atoms or electrons or stars, and because nursing is an interaction between humans, nursing research is concerned eventually with human populations, not populations of cells or atoms or electrons or stars. Research concerned with the practice of nursing is research concerned with the activities and responses of human beings, and the techniques of inquiry used when the population of interest is human are apt to be found in the scientific lore of the social rather than the natural sciences.

Any inquiry is a seeking, a search for something, for truth, for facts, for information, and it is what we do all the time in order to get the information we need to function. What is it that makes scientific inquiry different from this usual human activity?

Two characteristics differentiate scientific inquiry from the usual activities of information seeking: (1) scientific inquiry is always a *conscious* activity, and much information seeking is not conscious; and (2) explicit care is taken to avoid mistakes. How may the mistakes of human inquiry be avoided? By the use of what Babbie (1979) calls "scientific safeguards." These are things we do to make sure we are really observing what we think we are observing and reporting it the way it is. They are the activities of scientific inquiry.

When observation is a conscious act, using tested measurement devices, it tends to be more accurate. Selectivity and overgeneralization cannot easily occur if the specifics of observation (how many, what kind) are decided in advance and the observations are replicated, i.e., carried out again and again by the same or other observers. Scientific inquiry is a form of human inquiry, safeguarded in various ways to avoid error. The inquirer generally asks, and tries to answer, two questions: what is the pattern of events (what occurs) and why (what is the relationship between event A and event B that is responsible for the pattern)? The scientist wants not only to generate knowledge, but also to predict future events on the basis of that knowledge. Understanding *why* something happens increases the accuracy of the prediction.

STEPS IN THE RESEARCH PROCESS

The research process is how one carries out scientific, as opposed to human, inquiry. The framework for the process consists of three interactive phases: the conceptual phase, the empirical phase, and the interpretive phase (Kerlinger, 1973). In the conceptual phase, the boundaries of the problem and a focus for the study are identified, probably with the help of a literature review. Decisions are made as to what will be studied (the concepts and the variables) in which populations and how (data-collection techniques). Also considered at this time is how the information about the variables will be handled (data analysis). In the conceptual phase, the investigator decides what activities will be carried out in the empirical phase.

During the empirical phase, information is obtained that is relevant to the concepts and the variables, i.e., data are collected from the sample in accordance with the study design requirements. For our purposes in this chapter, *data* is defined as information gathered for research purposes.

Evaluation of the information, and perhaps prediction from it, constitutes the interpretive phase of the activity. The investigator examines the findings and determines what they mean.

This is a tidy framework for the steps of the research process. The key word in the framework, however, is *interactive*, which makes it somewhat less tidy. Conceptualization and interpretation continue during data collection, and information search and use is ever present. It is a mistake to believe that the phases occur in a natural and mutually exclusive sequence, along the lines of:

1. Think it all out (conceptual phase).
2. Go and do it (empirical phase).
3. See what it all means (interpretive phase).

In practice, the phases overlap in a spiral, rather than a linear, manner so that the usual form looks more like:

1. Think it all out—at the same time doing dry runs (pilot studies) and seeing what anyone else has done with the same or relevant concepts (literature review).
2. Go and do it—at the same time continuing with the

literature review, revising the technique of sample selection, reconceptualizing several of the variables, and doing early interpretation of the findings.

3. See what it all means—at the same time revising the concepts, dropping several variables, changing the plan for statistical evaluation, and planning the next study, which by now it will be obvious needs to be done.

The steps of the research process do not occur in a nice, neat sequence; they are, rather, a kind of gestalt, which is likely to be a little more organized than it appears to be while it is happening, but is certainly not so organized as it appears to be in the report of the study. It is probably incorrect to say that most investigators write the complete research design at the time they are writing up the findings for publication. It is probably correct to say that most investigators do not consider and carry out the steps in research strictly in the sequence presented here.

This book includes some of the basic rules for scientific inquiry; you read it in order that you may become a critical consumer of research. For this purpose, the steps in the research process are presented below in a logical chronology with a brief definition and description of each step. It is important to understand, however, that they seldom occur in such a tidy fashion.

Conceptual Phase

Defining the Problem. By defining the problem, you pull together in some organized way the whole set of factors, relationships, events, behaviors, whatever is giving you concern. Wandelt (1970) says that the problem is big—multifaceted, multivariable, too big for one study; many studies can be derived from one problem. The problem is the broad area of interest to the researcher. It provides the frame of reference for the study.

Literature Review. In the literature search, the investigator reviews the literature to see what other people have to say relevant to the problem. This helps to define more exactly the parameters of the proposed study. The literature considered may be either (a) theoretical, theories related to the content of the problem, or (b) empirical, reports of other studies that are relevant either to the content of the problem or to how it is addressed, the methodology.

Statement of the Purpose. The purpose is the focus of the study (Wandelt, 1970). It is the portion of the problem that the investigator wishes to consider. If hypotheses are stated, the purpose of the study is to test them. If research questions are asked, the purpose of the study is to answer them, so that the investigator may make a statement about the concepts represented by the variables in the question.

Identification of the Variables. The variables are those factors, or events or behaviors, about which information is desired.

Whatever they are, they may change as conditions change. Otherwise, they wouldn't be variables. Babbie (1979) defines variables as a set of mutually exclusive attributes. For instance, the variable *gender* has a set of mutually exclusive attributes called *Male* and *Female*. The attributes might also be called the *levels* of the variable.

Development of the Research Questions or Hypotheses. A *research question* is always (a) a question, (b) a question about relationships, (c) a question about relationships between or among variables. It indicates exactly what the investigator wants to find out in the study.

A hypothesis is always (for our purposes) (a) a statement, (b) a statement about relationships, (c) a statement about relationships between or among variables.

If the investigator does not know the probable answer, he asks the research question. If he thinks he knows the answers, he makes the statements, i.e., he predicts the relationship, he hypothesizes the relationship.

Identification of Types of Design. The research design reflects the intent of the investigator, who may be interested in exploration or description or in testing causal hypotheses. The methods of sample selection and data collection and analysis must reflect the intent. Methods appropriate to exploratory studies are not appropriate for testing causal hypotheses. The investigator's intent must be explicit so that the reader can evaluate the appropriateness of the design.

Identification of the Population. Populations are the people or events of interest to the investigator, the group that he wishes to say something about and from which he selects the sample.

You can see why it is so hard to talk about the steps in the research process one at a time. How can an investigator determine variables and ask research questions without having the population in mind? He probably took this step about the time he formulated the problem.

Sample Selection. The sample is the portion of the population that is studied in order to get information about the entire population. The assumption is that the sample can represent the population on the variables studied. The study findings derived from the sample are applied to the population from which the sample is selected.

Development of Data-Collection Strategies. This is the research plan: it indicates exactly what will be done with the sample in order to get the needed information and when, and what will be done with the information when it is obtained. In short, what will the investigator do, to whom, how, and how will the information obtained be analyzed?

Empirical Phase

Development of Data-Collection Instruments. Instruments (or tools) are things like questionnaires, observation schedules, and audit forms. The investigator must first find one, or make one, that will tell him what he needs to know and then test it. The instrument is not only a place to record information, but also dictates what information will be recorded. During the conceptual phase, the investigator figures out what that information should be and develops or finds an instrument that will obtain it. If the research question is about the relationship of diet to weight, the investigator needs a couple of instruments, one to get diet information and one to get weight scores. The diet instrument might consist of two questions, such as (1) do you eat only those foods allowed in your diet? (2) do you eat only those amounts allowed in your diet? There can be a group that answers both questions "yes" and a group that answers both questions "no." (There can also be a group that answers "yes" to question 1 and "no" to question 2, and a group that answers "no" to question 1 and "yes" to question 2.) Using the weight instrument (this will not have to be invented—it is called a scale), the investigator obtains the weight scores (the meter readings on the scale) for the groups. If the average weight loss for one group is different from the values for the other groups, then diet makes a difference to weight. Isn't research easy?

Fun maybe but not really easy. There are several reasons the diet instrument is not a good one. For one thing, the subjects are instructed to answer the questions either "yes" or "no." Maybe they would like to respond "sometimes," or "maybe," or "usually." Also, the investigator does not know whether the diet is really a weight loss diet or the subjects just think it is. Maybe calorie-counting questions would make a better instrument. Maybe a better design would be to have the investigator control the diet and assign samples from the population to different diet regimens. No matter what he does to improve the design, one source of error in the findings will always be present—the subjects may be fudging (no pun intended) on their diets and not reporting it.

The tools must be tested for reliability and validity. Is the instrument providing the desired information (validity), without fail (reliability)? The need for this testing is what puts the step of instrument development in the empirical phase, rather than in the conceptual phase.

Data Collection. When the instruments are ready and the sample is selected, the two are put together to collect data about the chosen variables. The investigator has thought heavily about all this in the conceptual phase, and now he just does what the design tells him to do. That's not really the way it works, of course. He is probably dealing with a sample of human subjects who have civil rights; even if the subjects are records, the data collectors are human. There are also the people he has to get past to have access to the subjects or the setting. The general law that holds is the usual one: anything that can go wrong will go wrong at the worst possible time. Therefore, the empirical phase always takes longer than planned.

Interpretive Phase

Data Analysis. Eventually, all the information is in place (or all the investigator is going to be able to get; at this stage, the study does not resemble the one put together in the conceptual phase). The time has come to analyze the data, which consists of breaking it into parts. There are two major steps: categorization and statistical analysis.

Categorization. A set of categories must be developed for each variable which will partition the responses according to some rule. The rule says which category gets which responses. For instance, if partitions for gender and religious belief are required, the categories for gender are probably going to be *Male* and *Female*. These will take care of the usual responses, although in terms of meaning exactly what you say, there are several biological levels of gender, and what is probably being recorded are secondary sex characteristics.

One of the rules about categories is that they have to include all the responses; there has to be a place to put all the information. If the categories for the partition of religious beliefs are *Catholic, Protestant, Jewish,* and *Other,* they will hold all the responses, but the agnostics and the atheists will be put in with the Hindus under *Other,* and the Methodists will be put in with the Episcopalians and the Baptists, under *Protestants.* Also, the categories will lump Roman Catholic and Greek Orthodox Catholic respondents together. The categories will accommodate all the responses, but they are not sensitive to some major differences in the respondents.

Statistical Analysis. The second step in data analysis includes some activities that we all know about, like counting (otherwise known as generating frequency distributions) and getting percentages and percentile ranks and finding the average of a set of scores and the range of the scores, and getting a numerical statement about the magnitude of a relationship between variables (coefficients of correlation). It also includes some activities that will not be covered in this book.

Interpretation of the Findings. Interpretation is the step in which the investigator tries to figure out what it all means. The analysis activity has provided a commodity called results, or findings. These results are usually numerical, frequently on the order of $t = 4.213$, $p < .05$; or $\bar{x} = 16.72$, $SD = 4$; or $\chi^2 = 6.04$, $p < .001$.

It is the responsibility of the researcher—the person who is taking all these steps in the research process—to do two things: translate the numbers into words and define what they mean. If the average score for group 1 is higher than that for group 2, does this mean that the members of group 1 are smarter than the members of group 2? Or better educated? Or more ethical? Do the findings support or take issue with some theory? Or some acknowledged fact? What is the meaning of a *t* test that is significant at the .05 level? Does the standard deviation suggest that the scores were clustered around the mean, or that they were far apart? If they were far apart, what does this indicate about the subjects? The investigator must do more than *report* the findings; he must *explain* them in terms of the problem and the purpose of the study.

Dissemination of the Findings

Publication is the final step in the process. The investigator must publish the work in some way (reading papers at conferences counts here but usually not very much) in order to lodge the findings in the literature. The last step taken by the researcher before he starts all over with new variables is to have the findings printed and become part of the literature about the old variables.

The purpose of this book is to help you understand the research process, so that you can criticize research design. The intent in criticism is not to find all the things the investigator did wrong, or did not do at all—although you may do this. Rather, it is to look at the technical soundness of the research process in order to decide whether the findings are acceptable to you as the products of good design, so that you may use them to make changes in your nursing care plan.

SUMMARY

Scientific inquiry is a form of *human inquiry* in which an explicit effort is made to avoid error. The steps in the research process are steps in scientific inquiry. The framework for the research process consists of three interactive phases: the *conceptual* phase, the *empirical* phase, and the *interpretive* phase. In the conceptual phase, the investigator defines the study *problem*, reviews the *relevant literature*, identifies the *purpose* of the study, identifies the relevant *variables*, develops *research questions* or *hypotheses*, decides which type of *design* is most appropriate, identifies a *population* and a *sample selection* process, and develops *data collection strategies*.

During the empirical phase, the investigator identifies or

develops data-collection *instruments* and uses them to collect the data from the sample in accordance with the dictates of the design.

During the interpretive phase, the investigator carries out data *analysis* and addresses the *meaning* of the findings in terms of the problem and the purpose of the study.

References

Babbie, E.R. The Practice of Social Research. Belmont, Calif.: Wadsworth, 1979.

Kerlinger, F.N. Foundations of Behavioral Research. 2d ed. New York: Holt, Rinehart & Winston, 1973.

Wandelt, M.A. Guide for the Beginning Researcher. New York: Appleton-Century-Crofts, 1970.

Study Activities

1. Use one or more of the definitions of *science* provided to indicate how nursing may be considered a science.

2. Describe the conceptual phase of the research process in terms of what steps the investigator takes in this phase, and why he takes them.

3. Describe the empirical phase of the research process in terms of what steps the investigator takes in this phase, and why he takes them.

4. An investigator is interested in knowing how level of education, years of experience, and type of care delivery are related to patient satisfaction. Write three research questions for this study. Using the same variables, write three hypotheses.

5. Differentiate human inquiry and scientific inquiry.

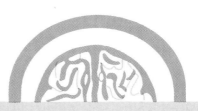

3

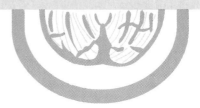

When you complete Chapter 3, you will be able to...

1. Differentiate theoretical frameworks from conceptual frameworks by
   a. Defining *theory*.
   b. Defining *conceptual framework*.

2. Discriminate levels of theory by
   a. Defining each of the three levels discussed.
   b. Explaining how they differ.

3. Describe the uses of theory.

4. Contrast *human* inquiry with *scientific* inquiry by
   a. Defining *human inquiry*.
   b. Defining *scientific inquiry*.
   c. Identifying the major differences in the definitions.

5. Distinguish the ways of knowing by
   a. Defining *agreement reality* and identifying likely sources of error.
   b. Defining *experiential reality* and identifying likely sources of error.

THEORY

THEORY AND CONCEPTUAL FRAMEWORKS

Science is logical and empirical; that is, it is concerned with both rationality and the observation of a real world of facts. A scientific understanding of the world must make logical sense and correspond to what is observed. For our purposes, we may say that theory deals with logic and research deals with the observation of facts. Theory describes logical relationships that are postulated by the theory to exist in the world; the research is designed to see whether the theoretical description of the world is correct, i.e., verified by the senses (Babbie, 1979).

Scientific philosophers do not agree as to the nature of theory, but we will follow the basic areas of agreement and let them continue their esoteric arguments without us.

Reynolds (1971), who has written a primer about theory, believes that theory provides a method of classifying and organizing data, the ability to predict (what happens to B if A is changed?), and the ability to explain (why and how did it happen, and what does it mean?). He says it can also provide a sense of understanding, although for most scientists, a sense of understanding is possible only when the *causal* mechanisms are described in the theory and tested.

Dubin (1969) differentiates between empirical systems and theoretical systems. An empirical system, he says, can be apprehended through human senses, but a theoretical system is constructed in the mind's eye to constitute a model, a representation, of reality. He suggests that a scientist tries to make the two systems congruent.

A useful definition of theory is found in an adaptation from Kerlinger (1964): *a theory will contain several propositions in general form, interrelated in certain ways, stated in such a way that it is possible to deduce specific testable hypotheses from the theory.* This definition tells you what a theory must contain in order to be a theory: *general propositions* that are *related* to one another and that allow the derivation of *testable hypotheses.*

According to Dubin (1969), the goals of science are prediction and understanding. For Kerlinger (1964), the basic aim of science is theory. They are in agreement, however, since Kerlinger believes that the basic aim of science is to find general explanations of events, and such general explanations are called theories.

In the dominant conceptions of theory, scientific knowledge is perceived as a set of well-supported empirical generalizations or laws, called *set-of-laws* theory, or as an interrelated set of definitions, axioms, and propositions. The latter, borrowed from mathematicians' conceptions of theory, is called *axiomatic* theory. Reynolds (1971) thinks that neither of these forms provides a sense of understanding, as this is usually given, although both forms can be used to derive explanations. In order for the sense of understanding to occur, a third theory, *causal process* theory, is required.

Theory may be classified in other ways, but this classification has the merit of including those many social science and nursing frameworks that are not yet subjected to rigorous testing.

It is necessary to the *generation* of theory to identify concepts and then use them in statements that purport to describe or explain reality. Concepts are the product of the classification and analysis of things studied. Dubin (1969) says that science deals with things, and in science, it is necessary to have a way of designating subject matter. As things are grouped together, concepts form. However, a collection of concepts of a discipline's subject matter does not constitute the discipline's theory. As concepts are put together, theories emerge to present models of the world. Concepts are mental abstracts.

Theories have both existence statements, which claim the existence of the phenomenon referred to by a concept, and relational statements, which describe the relationships between the concepts. Definitions describe concepts; existence statements claim they exist. Relational statements indicate that knowledge about one concept conveys information about another concept (Reynolds, 1971). These statements may claim associations (A is related to B on Tuesdays but not on Thursdays) or causation (A causes B on Tuesdays but not on Thursdays).

In *testing* theories, the concern is with the degree of correspondence between the theoretical statements and the empirical data, i.e., what is apprehended in the real world by the senses. It is usually not possible to examine simultaneously the correspondence between data and all the statements that constitute a theory. Most theory-testing research is designed to provide evidence for the usefulness of one theoretical concept, or maybe a few concepts. However, *direct* support from the data for one theoretical statement provides *indirect* support for all the statements in the theory.

Theories are used to explain or predict phenomena. The correct question is not which theory is right or wrong, but which provides the most comprehensive explanation of the phenomena of interest. One is never interested in the "truth" of the theory, since science concerns itself with accurate description and plausible explanation of phenomena, not a search for "truth." The theory is interesting because of its usefulness for prediction and explanation.

No single empirical study can provide enough evidence to reject a theory completely. Immediate, complete rejection is usually not the intent, although some philosophers suggest that science only advances as theories are destroyed to make room for new and better theories (Dubin, 1969). Whether or not this point of view is accepted, theory testing is likely to be piecemeal. If a theory is considered to be a set of descriptions of causal processes, it will define the conditions under which the processes occur. It is effective to ask how much impact a process has under certain conditions (on Tuesday rather than on Thursday, for instance), rather than which one is *the* causative process. If we know that A causes B on Tuesday, we can specify what happens on Tuesday and worry about Thursday later.

Theories and other scientific statements can be compared on two characteristics: precision and generality. Precision refers to the accuracy of the prediction, and generality refers to the range of different situations to which a theory can be applied.

Abstract statements (theoretical concepts) cannot be proved, although they may, with some effort, be disproved. Concrete statements can be determined to be true or false: the event occurred or it did not. The concrete statements provide *indirect* support for the abstract statements; that is, testing hypotheses about the relationship between facts, when the predicted relationships are based in theory, allows the theory itself to be tested. As abstract statements are found to be useful descriptions of more and more situations, confidence in the statements increases, and the theory becomes acceptable as an explanation for a set of events, or as a basis for practice.

Even the most precise and widely accepted definitions can be used only to organize or classify data; they cannot be used for prediction or explanation or to provide a sense of understanding. Only when the *relationship* statements are developed can these goals be obtained (Reynolds, 1971). The distinction is particularly important in nursing because it *may* be that theories in nursing are elaborated sets of concepts, with little elaboration of the relationship between the concepts. Or it *may not* be so. The point is that without the development and exploration of the relationship statements, the theory cannot provide a basis for practice. The educated nurse, therefore, examines the various nursing theories critically and continually.

Such examination suggests that the theories and conceptual models in nursing exist at various levels of abstractness and comprehensiveness (Fitzpatrick and Whall, 1983), and it is not always clear how they may be used to guide nursing practice. Whether the same practice decisions will be made in a nursing situation by nurses practicing out of different theoretical models needs to be considered.

In their description of their model for theory development in nursing, Chinn and Jacobs (1978) say that theory development is the most crucial task in nursing and that unless research is undertaken with the aim of incorporation into theory, findings are likely to remain a compilation of isolated facts. Many years earlier, Merton (1957) was addressing a similar issue in sociology and came to the same conclusion: The researchers must learn to work with the theorists in order that the discipline knowledge contained in an enormous aggregate of facts can be organized and explained.

Theories "constitute the mechanisms by which researchers organize empirical findings into a meaningful pattern" (Polit and Hungler, 1983, p. 98). They allow the investigator to predict what will happen (by way of hypothesis) and even explain why.

Theories are, by nature, very structured. They require, at the least, definitions of concepts and a set of statements that indicate the relationships among the concepts. The theory must provide a mechanism for the logical derivation of new statements from old ones (Polit and Hungler, 1983).

Polit and Hungler (1983) differentiate theoretical frameworks from conceptual frameworks: conceptual frameworks are less formal, less well-developed attempts to organize phenomena and may lack the system of statements of relationships between concepts that allows progress to new statements.

A theory is more than a lot of ideas strung together; there are some rules about what is required before one speaks of having a theory. Although conceptual frameworks may be a little less structured, they must still be more than a free association of ideas in written form.

Science is open-ended. No theory is expected to be eternal, and any fact or set of facts may be changed by new knowledge.

For theorists and researchers this is a way of life; if one's theory is wiped out by new knowledge, one must rethink and try again. A wiped-out theory is not necessarily a "bad" theory. When a more *usable* theory, one that explains more facts with less effort, is developed, an older, less explanatory framework must be reconsidered, and perhaps abandoned.

WAYS OF KNOWING

Human knowledge may be organized and elaborated in theoretical and conceptual frameworks. But where does it come from in the first place? Fundamentally, knowledge is whatever most people agree is so, most of the time. Babbie (1979) identifies *agreement reality* and *experiential reality* as ways of knowing: you know things are real because you have been told they are real by authorities in agreement with one another; or you know things are real because you have experienced them.

Knowledge in nursing and other sciences is based partly on a general agreement as to what is so and partly on what can be observed, i.e., experienced. Agreement about what is so has a tendency to grow out of *tradition*; we do not need to inquire because we accept what we all know. The difficulty is that what we all know may be wrong: for example, we all knew for years that after a normal delivery, a primipara must be kept on bed rest for 2 weeks. However, when World War II depleted the nursing staff in civilian hospitals, primiparas were getting out of bed within several hours of delivery and have continued to do so without adverse effects.

Authority is another source of knowledge by agreement: we tend to trust the judgment of people with special expertise. Although they may be in error on any given point, we not only trust them in their own fields, but also expect them to be authorities in other fields. Two examples immediately come to mind: the athletes on television who are able to identify the best razor or the best beer because they can throw a football and the physicians who are considered qualified to give advice about nursing problems, or anything else in hospital life, because they understand medical problems.

Although it is frequently a mistake to accept knowledge based on agreement (and, of course, frequently *not* a mistake), experience is not a perfect source of information either. Observations of the events about which one is seeking knowledge may be inaccurate, and what is perceived is not what occurred. Observations may be selective; that is, the observer has a hunch that a certain event, or pattern of events, exists and looks for things to observe that support the hunch, meanwhile ignoring everything else. An observer may observe accurately enough and then overgeneralize; that is, she may observe a few events and then decide that that is how it always is.

Research methodology is a special approach to the discovery of reality through experience (Babbie, 1979). As you begin to understand the steps in the research process, you will see that they are taken in a conscious effort to inhibit or avoid the errors inherent in the search for knowledge through experience.

SUMMARY

Theories contain *interrelated propositions* in general form, from which *testable hypotheses* may be derived. Theories are used to *explain* and *predict* phenomena.

Conceptual frameworks are less formal, less well-developed explanatory frameworks, which may lack the relational components of theory.

Ways of knowing are discussed in terms of the characteristics of *agreement reality* (you know things are real because you have been told they are real by authorities in agreement) and *experiential reality* (you know things are real because you have experienced them). Research methodology is a special form of experiential reality.

References

Babbie, E.R. The Practice of Social Research. 2d ed. Belmont, Calif.: Wadsworth, 1979.

Chinn, P.L., and M.K. Jacobs. A model for theory development in nursing. In P.L. Chinn (ed.). Advances in Nursing Science. Germantown, MD: Aspen, 1978, pp. 1–11.

Dubin, R. Theory Building. New York: Free Press, 1969.

Fitzpatrick, J.J., and A.L. Whall. Conceptual Models of Nursing: Analysis and Application. Bowie, MD: Robert J. Brady, 1983.

Kerlinger, F.N. Foundations of Behavioral Research. New York: Holt, Rinehart & Winston, 1964.

Merton, R.K. Social Theory and Social Structure. Revised. New York: Free Press, 1957.

Polit, D., and B. Hungler. Nursing Research: Principles and Methods. 2d ed. Philadelphia: J.B. Lippincott, 1983.

Reynolds, P. A Primer in Theory Construction. New York: Bobbs-Merrill, 1971.

Study Activities

1. Differentiate a conceptual framework from a theory.

2. Differentiate the three levels of theory presented in the text in terms of their structure and use.

3. Differentiate agreement reality and experiential reality in terms of the source of the knowledge base.

4. Using the definition of theory provided in the text, determine whether your nursing curriculum is theory-based. Defend your decision by indicating what is contained in the model that makes it a theory, or what the model requires to make it a theory.

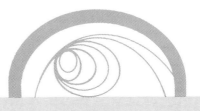

4

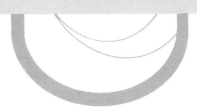

When you complete Chapter 4, you will be able to...

1. Distinguish among *problem, purpose,* and *research question* and *hypothesis* by
   a. Demonstrating the relationship between problem and purpose.
   b. Demonstrating the relationship between purpose and research question and/or hypothesis.

2. Differentiate *research question* from *hypothesis* by
   a. Defining and writing research questions.
   b. Defining and writing hypotheses.
   c. Explaining the difference and the basis of the difference.

3. Differentiate *variable* from *concept* by
   a. Defining *variable.*
   b. Defining *concept.*
   c. Explaining the relationship between the two definitions.

4. Differentiate *independent variable* from *dependent variable* by
   a. Defining *independent variable* and indicating how an assigned independent variable differs from an active independent variable.
   b. Defining *dependent variable.*
   c. Explaining the relationship between an independent variable and a dependent variable.

5. Explain *operational definition* by
   a. Defining a measured operational definition.
   b. Defining an experimental operational definition.
   c. Demonstrating the relationship between the two.
   d. Indicating why operational definitions of variables are important to research.

DEFINING THE PROBLEM

PROBLEM TO PURPOSE

The word *problem*, like the word *science*, has several meanings. The idea of "something to resolve" is there, perhaps with negative overtones. It is difficult to define the word exactly. For instance:

1. A task in arithmetic is called a problem.
2. Patients have problems that may or may not be nursing problems.
3. Nurses have problems that may or may not be related to patient problems.
4. Nursing practice problems are different from either nurses' problems or patients' problems and may be clinical or organizational.

In research, the word may have a different meaning from any of these. Authors are not in agreement as to the meaning of the word, although they all agree that whatever the meaning, the problem should be clearly formulated (Babbie, 1979; Brink and Wood, 1983; Kerlinger, 1973; Polit and Hungler, 1983; Wandelt, 1970).

Brink and Wood (1983), for instance, in explaining why clear formulation of the problem is so important, tell us that it provides the frame of reference for the entire study, structures the ideas of the researcher, and dictates the content of the literature review.

Gay (1976) says that the problem identifies a broad area of interest, which is in some way related to the area of expertise of the investigator. This definition supports the way this word is used in the book, following Wandelt (1970, p. 1), who perceives the problem as the "irritation that stimulates interest and prompts investigation." It is complex, an entity too large to be the subject of a single investigation. The definition of a problem identifies and describes many elements and their various facets. A problem is always multifaceted, of global proportions, and difficult to define in a single sentence.

Where are problems found? They are found where Brink and Wood (1983) find what they call research topics; they say that such topics are based in thoughts, observations, experiences, and arise out of an area of knowledge. A problem is found in the same places. It contains research topics, and indeed, several research topics may be generated from one problem, as Wandelt (1970) uses the word *problem*.

The purpose of a study is more explicit than the problem. It is derived from the problem and focuses on the particular elements of the problem to be studied. Wandelt (1970, p. 4) says: "... the definition of problem will identify and describe the many elements and their various facets of which the problem is composed. The statement of purpose will identify one particular set of elements of the problem about which new knowledge will be sought. Distinguishing between the two terms in this way reminds us also that the goal of research is not the solution of particular problems, but, rather, the revelation of new knowledge."

Let us look at a problem, keeping in mind that it is multifaceted, composed of related concepts, and use it to develop a few statements of purpose. The statement of purpose is the statement of the focus of the study; it identifies the elements from the problem that are selected for consideration. Suppose that a nurse named John Alden (his name is John Alden because he is going to speak for himself in his problem formulation) uses Orem's Theory of Self-Care as a framework for his practice. As a staff nurse on an oncology unit, he is subject to the bureaucratic structure of the institution; he does not control staffing or medical perceptions and decisions or patient conditions. To help him develop his practice, he reads articles in clinical journals in nursing and in other fields. The articles, written by psychologists, sociologists, pastors and supervisory nurses, describe nursing responsibilities to dying patients, and he is informed that he should spend time with dying patients, talk with them about the fact that they are dying, and assist the patients' families in their grief work. Although he is inclined to agree with the statements in the literature, it is his experience that on 3 days out of 7, staffing is such that he is responsible for 15 patients, 7 of whom are terminal and 2 of whom are comatose; the physicians on the unit usually do not tell dying patients the medical prognosis;

and families are conspicuous by their absence. He begin
wonder how useful all those studies are to his nursing care pl
He formulates a problem that looks like this:

The constraints on nursing time and nurses' behavior impoᵥᵤu
by organization policy and health system power hierarchies are
not addressed realistically in nursing literature. Also, while the
nursing function certainly requires command of psychosocial and
managerial as well as technical skills, it should be somewhat less
than all encompassing. There is no doubt that nurses have
responsibilities to and for the dying patient which are not always
met, but those responsibilities may not differ greatly from their
responsibilities to all patients in their care. The need to identify
self-care deficits and establish nursing systems as appropriate
may be related to medical diagnosis but surely should be independent of medical prognosis.*

Several research studies can be found in this problem, and
the investigator must decide which one he wishes to focus on.
John Alden is interested in organization primarily as it affects
his patient-care activities. He might choose to focus on whether
there is a difference in nursing responsibility or nursing behavior
when the patient is considered terminal. Do the nursing acts
change when the patient is labeled terminal, or are the activities
of identifying self-care deficits and establishing nursing systems
the same for terminal and nonterminal patients? Because his
interests are clinical, he decides to focus his research on the
clinical variables. Using the concepts he formulated in the problem, he might state a study purpose: the purpose of this study is
to determine the relationship between nursing interventions and
medical prognosis. Or he could say: the purpose of this study is
to test the hypothesis that nurses spend less time talking with
patients who are dying than they spend with patients who are
not dying. Or, if he wishes to test the constructs of Orem's theory,
the purpose of the study could be to determine the relationship
between the number of self-care deficits identified and the medical prognosis. Each of these study purposes comes from one or
two of the concepts formulated in the problem; the purposes are
related to the problem in that they are based in problem concepts.
All the problem concepts, however, are not found in any one of
the studies, since the purpose identifies only the portion of the
problem that is to be considered.

*Freely adapted with permission from M.R. Castles and
R.B. Murray, *Dying in an Institution: Nurse Patient Per-
spectives* (New York: Appleton-Century-Crofts, 1979), p.1.
Copyright 1979 by Appleton-Century-Crofts.

The head nurse on the oncology unit (her name is Priscilla Mullins, because she wishes her nurses to continue to speak for themselves) is probably more interested in the organizational constraints mentioned in the problem formulation. If she does a study, the focus might be on the effects of staffing patterns on time spent with patients, and her statement of purpose might be: the purpose of this study is to determine whether there is more sustained interaction with patients when the staff consists of registered nurses only than when there is a professional/non-professional mix.

As you can see from this example, many studies can be developed from one problem. The investigator should make clear which problem concepts are addressed in the study; it is against the rules to formulate a problem and then state a purpose that has no clear relationship to any of the problem concepts. If Priscilla Mullins, having formulated the problem, stated that the purpose of her study was to identify the impact of staffing patterns on patient satisfaction with care, research eyebrows would be raised. One of her major concepts (patient satisfaction with care) is not present in the problem formulation; the question would arise as to why she studies satisfaction, when there is nothing in her formulation of the problem to suggest that satisfaction is related to anything.

The purpose must always indicate the focus of the study. It is specific, but it may be more or less comprehensive. For example, according to Brink and Wood (1983), the purpose must indicate exactly what the investigator intends to do to answer the questions. It should include how data are to be collected or what is observed, the setting of the study, and the subjects of the study. Gay (1976) writes about a "specific researchable problem" that will indicate the variables of interest and the relationships to be investigated; Polit and Hungler (1983, p. 71) conceptualize the "statement of the research problem" in similar terms. These definitions are analogous to the Wandelt (1970) "statement of purpose."

Gay (1976) believes that the specific researchable problem should be accompanied by the presentation of background material that justifies the study in terms of the problem's significance. Such background is necessary to understand the problem. Her "background material" probably contains Wandelt's "definition of the problem"; in that framework, it will precede the statement of purpose, the statement of the "specific researchable problem."

Authors agree on important points, like the necessity for a clear formulation of a set of broad concepts of interest to the researcher. This must precede a more specific identification of the focus of an individual study, a focus that will be derived from the set of broad concepts. The language varies a little, but there is agreement on the basic concepts. Wandelt's language on this subject is used in the book.

The statement of purpose is derived from the formulation of the problem and always indicates the focus of the study. It may or may not state the data collection techniques that will be used or identify populations. It always names the variables of interest, although they may be identified at an abstract level. For instance, the purpose of the study may be to identify the effect of anxiety on performance. Although the abstract concepts must be stated as measurable variables at some time, it need not be done in the statement of the purpose.

VARIABLES AND CONCEPTS

In the preceding section, two important terms have been used without any attempt to define them: *variables* and *concepts*. You probably know in a general way what they mean, but in order to be a critical reader of research, it is necessary to understand the terms more exactly.

Babbie (1979) tackles the definition of variable by first defining *attributes*: these are characteristics or qualities that describe an object. Any descriptive statement involves an attribute: for instance, the tree is *green*; the patient is *agitated*; the man is a *bookkeeper*; half the subjects in the experiment are *female*. The italicized words are attributes, and variables are logical groupings of attributes. *Male* and *female* are attributes: Gender is the variable comprising these two attributes. Another way to look at it is to say that attributes are levels of a variable. The levels of the variable Social Class—the attributes of the subjects—are probably something like *upper class*, *middle class*, and *lower class*. In the problem formulated by John Alden, the variable Medical Prognosis has two levels, two attributes of the subjects: *terminal* and *nonterminal*. The variable Nursing Behavior in the Alden–Mullins studies probably consists of the attributes *spends time with patients* and *does not spend time with patients*.

There can be more than two attributes, but there must be at least two, since a variable is a set of mutually exclusive attributes. If everyone in the population of interest to the investigator is female, Gender is not a variable; rather, it is a constant in that population.

A variable is a general class or category of objects, events, or situations; within this general class, specific examples of the class vary (Cozby, 1981). Gay (1976) says that a variable is a concept that can assume any one of a range of values. Polit and Hungler (1983) also define it in terms of concepts—as concepts that are operationalized, abstract entities that take on different values. You may be starting to think that you were better off with a less exact understanding of the word.

You really are not, but it is understandable that you might think so. Take a deep breath and let it out slowly. Because variable is defined by way of concept, you must consider the meaning of concept. Polit and Hungler (1983) remind us that research is concerned with abstract phenomena; abstractions are referred to as concepts. The concepts are not directly measurable, and in order to study them, they must be translated into variables, which are measurable. A concept may be identified in a word or a phrase symbolizing several related ideas (Brink and Wood, 1983). Anxiety is a concept; quality of nursing care is a concept; and patient satisfaction, self-care deficit, and therapeutic intervention are all concepts.

Babbie (1979) is a sociologist by profession, and he is interested in the "existence" of *prejudice*; he concludes that despite a good many sociological studies purporting to measure prejudice, it has no real existence. It cannot be seen or heard or smelled or touched or tasted. What does exist is behaviors, experiences, observations, and a *mental image* of what those behaviors, experiences, and observations represent, what they have in common. Mental images cannot be communicated (or measured), and in order to communicate about them, we need to agree about how they *should* look. We come to some agreement about what the terms used to describe the mental images mean, and then we begin to shape our own mental images to correspond to the general agreement. The correspondence is never perfect. No two persons have the *same* mental images, although common factors are shared for any given mental image.

Another term for mental image is *concept*. You already know that a concept is abstract and cannot be measured. So why are there instruments designed to measure the concept of *prejudice*? Although in human inquiry it is possible to obtain useful information on the basis of vague and general agreement about the meaning of terms, in scientific inquiry we must specify exactly what we "mean." This specification of meaning is what must be done to communicate about concepts and measure them. The investigator who wants to examine the *concept* of prejudice must specify the *indicators* of prejudice. The indicators are real; they are observable phenomena taken to indicate the presence or absence of prejudice.

In order to measure a concept, it is necessary to specify one or more observable events that indicate its presence. If Dr. Smith writes an order stating that his patients must not be assigned to nurse John Alden for bedside care, he will be foolish and perhaps be sued. If he quietly suggests to the head nurse that he would prefer that John Alden not be assigned to his patients, and that he would be grateful if that could be managed, the legal action is less likely, but the behavior is equally indicative of "prejudice against male nurses." The behavior is real; it can be identified and counted. It is an indicator. It is an *operational definition* of prejudice.

Along with indicators, concepts have dimensions: the concept of *compassion*, for instance, may have feeling dimensions (John Alden does not like to see Mrs. Brown in pain) and action dimensions (he asks the surgeon for a p.r.n. pain medication). Specifying the dimensions and the collection of indicators for each dimension is how we can define and measure the concept (Babbie, 1979).

The definition of the concept does not purport to give the "real" meaning of anything. It simply focuses the investigator on two things: *what* must be observed to say anything about the concept and *how* the observations must be carried out.

Now, think about the definitions of variable presented earlier: a concept that can assume a range of values, concepts operationalized. Anxiety is a concept, and an important one in nursing. All kinds of things may be associated with anxiety, and nurses would like to find out if they are. But the concept of anxiety cannot be observed; behaviors are observed, and when certain groups of behaviors are present, the inference is made that anxiety is present. Suppose an investigator puts together a test based on those behaviors, called the Smith Anxiety Scale, and gets agreement that the scale measures the concept. (It is not as easy to agree to that as you might think, but let us save that for later.) Then he has a variable, an operationalized concept, that can assume a range of values, say, from 1 to 50. A subject could score any place on the scale. The name of the concept is anxiety; the name of the variable is really the score on the Smith Anxiety Scale, but the investigator is likely to name it after the concept and call it anxiety. The difference between the variable and the concept is that the variable can be measured and different values can be obtained in the population of interest. Getting the different population values just means that the investigator gives the Smith Anxiety Scale to the subjects and determines whether a subject is anxious or not on the basis of the test score. At the least, the investigator can say that the subject scored 30 on the scale, and since the other subjects made other scores, whatever concept the scale really measures, it is a variable. The levels of the variable are the scores on the test.

Another word you will encounter in research reports is *construct*. Investigators tend to use the words *concept* and *construct* interchangeably (Polit and Hungler, 1983). Those who do not are making differentiations we do not need: for our purpose, concept and construct are synonymous.

Investigators may want to know more than the fact that variables are associated; they probably want to know how. Does variable A *influence* variable B, or do they just occur together in some regular pattern? When the question arises of which is an influencing variable in a set of variables, it becomes necessary to refine the earlier general definition of a variable and define an *independent* variable and a *dependent* variable.

Independent variables are frequently defined as presumed causes, as stimuli, as influencers. They are *manipulated* by the investigator, who wishes to study the effect of the manipulation on the dependent variables. Dependent variables change as a result of changes in the independent variables. They are dependent on independent variables. If the independent variable is the stimulus, the dependent variable is the response (Babbie, 1979; Brink and Wood, 1983; Gay, 1976; Polit and Hungler, 1983). Variation in the dependent variable reflects the variation in the independent variable; that is, as the investigator manipulates the independent variable, measurable changes occur in the dependent variable. Note that the dependent variable is *not* under the control of the investigator, except as he is able to manipulate the independent variable.

For instance, John Alden may want to know whether spending time listening to terminal patients makes them more comfortable. He may think that the nursing intervention of *listening to the patient for one-half hour a day* results in increased patient comfort, such that the need for narcotic analgesics decreases. He can hypothesize that the specified nursing intervention *listening* influences patient comfort so that an experimental group exposed to the intervention requires less medication for pain than a control group not exposed to the intervention.

The nursing intervention is his independent variable, and it has two levels: offered and not offered. One group of subjects (note that the patients have become subjects, since Alden is applying the intervention for research purposes, not clinical purposes) gets the intervention every day for 3 months. The other group does not. Alden **manipulates** the independent variable by offering or not offering the nursing treatment. He does so to see if the manipulation of the independent variable affects the dependent variable, amount of drug use. He measures the dependent variable by determining the amount of narcotic analgesic used by each subject. If one group uses a lesser amount during the specified time, he may make a cautious statement about the influence of the independent variable, the nursing intervention, on the dependent variable, patient comfort as measured by the amount of narcotic analgesic used.

Variables are not inherently independent or dependent (Polit and Hungler, 1983); they are defined as such by the investigator. Babbie (1979) gives us an example. If an investigator is interested in knowing whether women are more religious than men (the hypothesis is that religiosity is a function of gender), the independent variable is gender and the dependent variable is religiosity. In another study, or even another part of the same study, when the analysis is concerned with the impact of religiosity on crime, religiosity may be the independent variable and crime rate, the dependent variable.

If the investigator is not interested in causation, or in the direction of an influence, but only wishes to know whether the two variables are associated, there is no need to identify variables as independent or dependent. They are all equally variables together; which influences the other is not addressed. However, investigators need not be interested in causality to be identifying independent and dependent variables; they may only be interested in knowing the direction of the influence of one variable on another. An investigator who finds that women are less likely to report themselves as being risk takers than are men can suggest that gender influences attitudes toward risk taking. Gender is considered to be the independent variable and attitudes, the dependent variable, since that is obviously the direction of the influence. Hardly anyone is likely to believe that attitudes influence gender. The researcher would not, however, be so foolish as to say that gender *causes* attitudes toward risk taking, only that the association exists.

If the researcher wants to know whether nursing intervention resulted in beneficent outcomes in patients, the serenity of a mere study of association cannot be his. He must say that one variable influences another variable, and which one influences the other. Because the researcher would rather not think that patient outcomes cause nursing interventions, the interventions will be defined as the independent variable.

Given that the investigator knows which variable is which and needs to define them for the study, he will need to consider two more terms associated with independent variables: an *active* independent variable is one that the investigator can actually manipulate; an *assigned* independent variable cannot be manipulated, but is assigned the status of independent variable by the investigator. Investigators do not usually mention active and assigned independent variables in their reports, but you need to be able to identify them.

In a study to examine the impact of reinforcement on learning, reinforcement is an *active* independent variable. The investigator may use reward techniques to reinforce one group of learners and punishment techniques to reinforce another group of learners, in order to see which group learns the most. The variable of reinforcement is actually manipulated: sometimes he rewards, sometimes he punishes. In the same study, gender may be an *assigned* independent variable. The investigator assigns gender the status of independent variable in the study. The purpose may be to determine whether men learn more than women in reward rather than punishment situations. The variable of gender cannot be manipulated by having people sometimes be men and sometimes be women, but the investigator can certainly put the learning scores for men in one column and the learning scores for women in another column and see which group has the best average, the best mean score for the group. He uses a statistical technique (comparing the mean scores of the two groups) to "manipulate" the independent variable of gender. He must, by the way, be sure that his assigned independent variable precedes his dependent variable. If he cannot make the case that one obviously precedes the other, he does not have an assigned independent variable. Organismic variables (e.g., age, gender, medical diagnosis) and demographic variables (e.g., income, social class, level of education) are frequently assigned the status of independent variables. They cannot be manipulated by the investigator, but they can be handled using sampling or statistical techniques.

FORMULATING RESEARCH QUESTIONS AND HYPOTHESES

Now that you know about variables, you need to learn what to do with them. You use them to ask research questions or to state hypotheses. Both research questions and hypotheses are concerned with *relationships*, relationships between or among variables.

The obvious difference between a research question and a hypothesis is that the research question is a question and the hypothesis is a declarative sentence. The less obvious difference is in what the investigator must know to formulate one or the other. Both forms express an interest in examining or establishing relationships between variables. If there is little information about whether there is a relationship, the investigator asks the research question. If he has a hunch, or a theory, or can make an educated guess based in some observations, he makes the hypothesis.

The research question is a question about the relationship between *two or more* variables. It must contain at least two variables. If the charge nurse on a unit asks, "Why is staff morale so low?" that is not a research question because there is only one variable (staff morale). It is a perfectly good administrative question, and he would like the answer, but he cannot get the answer by using the research process. Research is concerned with relationships. If the charge nurse would say, "Staff morale is certainly low. I wonder if there is some relationship between the nurses' morale and the staff-patient ratio. Or maybe they are unhappy because they have to punch the time clock," he would be on the right track and beginning to think like an investigator. He is asking, "What is the relationship between staff morale and staff-patient ratios?" and "What is the relationship between staff morale and personnel policy?" He could answer those questions, using the research process. If he had a hunch about what the relationships might be, he could state some hypotheses. "It is hypothesized that there is a positive relationship between staff morale and good staffing patterns," or "There is a relationship between morale and personnel policies such that factory-based personnel policies (time clocks) result in low staff morale." He could design a study to test the hypotheses. Testing hypotheses means seeing if the predicted relationships exist in the way that the hypotheses say they do.

On the whole, it is better for the investigator to make hypotheses, if he can, than to ask research questions. Polit and Hungler (1983, p. 134) correctly point out that "initial efforts to investigate phenomena are usually strengthened by the formulation of hypotheses." They add that any time there is a relationship, there is a potential hypothesis, and the investigator has nothing to lose by developing predictions about the relationship. It is possible to make a stronger case for research questions in exploratory and descriptive studies, where the investigator may not have enough information about the variables to make plausible predictions, and they mention this. If predictions are made too early, investigators may become so enamored of the hypotheses that they do not wish to give them up; if they make them too soon, the parting may be painful. It might be easier all around to ask research questions during exploratory and descriptive work and *then* state and test hypotheses. The fact remains, however, that if hypotheses are not made and tested, the science does not develop (Kerlinger, 1973; Polit and Hungler, 1983). Sometimes the choice between the question and the statement is simply a matter of personal style.

The hypothesis states an expected relationship between variables and should define the variables in measurable terms (Gay, 1976; Polit and Hungler, 1983). It may be stated in abstract terms, but since it must be testable, it is commonly stated in terms of some kind of measurement (for instance, scores on a test) or of statistical differences (the mean of Group A will be greater than the mean of Group B).

The prediction can be one of association (anxiety is related to stress) or of difference (the anxiety scores of Group A will be greater than the anxiety scores of Group B). The prediction may or may not have a direction. The investigator may say that A is positively related to B (i.e., high on A, high on B; low on A, low on B) or that A is inversely related to B (i.e., high on A, low on B; low on A, high on B). If differences are predicted, the prediction may be that A is greater than B or that A is less than B.

The investigator may want to play it a little safer, and not predict the direction of the relationship. In this case, he would say only that A is related to B, or that A is different from B. If direction is predicted, he may be wrong in two ways: in the fact of the relationship (or difference) and in the direction of the relationship (or difference). Despite the possibility of error, the direction of the expected association or difference is a useful part of the hypothesis. For instance, it is no help to know that the amount of time nurses spend with patients is related to patient satisfaction with care unless it is also known whether high satisfaction results from a greater amount of time spent, or a lesser amount of time spent.

Sometimes, in making hypotheses, the investigator will make the null hypothesis, which is really not useful, since the null hypothesis is what the statistic will test anyhow. The null hypothesis is the hypothesis of no difference, or more exactly, it is the hypothesis that population means are equal and the observed difference in the sample is due to random error. The research hypothesis (sometimes called the alternative hypothesis) predicts that population means are not equal and that the observed difference is due to the effect of the independent variable (Cozby, 1981). The research hypothesis is what the investigator really thinks is so and he might as well say it. The statistic tests the null; if the independent variable made enough difference to be perceptible to the statistic, then the researcher rejects the null hypothesis and accepts (very carefully and hedging his bets) the research hypothesis; if the investigator is able to reject the null, the research hypothesis is supported.

The best place for the purpose and the research questions or hypotheses to occur is after the literature review. This simplifies for the reader the task of determining that the purpose is derived from the broader problem, and that the variables in the research questions or hypotheses reflect both the statement of purpose and the broader concepts formulated in the problem, as these are inferred from the literature review.

OPERATIONAL DEFINITIONS

Operational definitions of variables remove ambiguity from the meanings assigned to variables and allow other investigators to replicate studies. If one researcher finds in one population that nurses avoid terminal patients, that is only interesting. If 15 investigators find the same thing when they carry out the same study in other populations, it begins to support a relationship between medical prognosis and the behavior of nurses. But unless the 15 other investigators know exactly what the first investigator "means by" avoidance, replication is impossible. An operational definition of a variable assigns meaning to the variable by specifying the activities, the "operations" necessary to measure the variable. This is not as easy as it sounds. You might be considering, while you read, what an operational definition of professional nursing care would look like.

Kerlinger (1973, p. 30) believes that a word can be defined in two ways: by using other words and by saying what actions or behaviors the word expresses. The variable *intelligence* may be defined as *mental acuity*, using other words. It may also be defined by telling what actions or behaviors are carried out to measure the variable, for example, intelligence is the score on the Smith Mental Test.

An operational definition assigns meaning to a variable by specifying the operations necessary to measure the variable or by specifying how the investigator manipulates the variable. If an investigator wants to replicate a study, the replication is easier, and more reliable, if he has operational definitions of the variables. It is simpler to get Smith Mental Test scores than to come to some agreement as to the meaning of mental acuity.

There are two kinds of operational definitions: measured operational definitions and experimental operational definitions. A *measured operational definition* is one that describes how a variable will be measured. For instance, staff nurse achievement may be measured by patient satisfaction, supervisor rating, or a checklist of tasks accomplished. An *experimental operational definition* spells out the way an investigator will manipulate the independent variable. In a study of the impact of reinforcement on learning, reward might be operationally defined as praising an effort and punishment might be operationally defined as blaming the subject for not doing more. The definition would include what the investigator did to reward and what he did to blame (Kerlinger, 1973, p. 31).

Operational definitions as such are not usually found in the research literature. It is more common practice for the investigator to mention the variables of the study early in the research report and in a later section, discuss the instruments used to measure the variables, or discuss the experimental procedures used to manipulate the independent variables. In a good explanation of the methodology of data collection, the variables are operationally defined.

The benefit of operational definitions is that they facilitate communication among investigators; operational definitions are not subject to misinterpretation of meaning. However, they do not describe all the meaning there is in a variable. The "meaning" of intelligence is not entirely described by the Smith Mental Test. The operational definition enables scientists to talk with one another without ambiguity and replicate one another's studies, but we all understand that we "mean" more than the operations allow. Are you ready to develop an operational definition of professional nursing care?

SUMMARY

A clearly formulated *problem* identifies a *broad area of interest* to the investigator. It is *complex, multivariable,* and contains topics for several studies.

The statement of the *purpose* identifies the *focus of the study*. It is *derived* from the *problem* and indicates the *concepts* or *variables* about which new knowledge will be sought in a particular study.

A *concept* is an abstract phenomenon that is not directly measurable. A *variable* is a phenomenon that can be *measured*; the investigator measures the variable with the understanding that the variable represents the concept.

The study *variables* are presented in *research questions* or *hypotheses*. A research question is a question about relationships among variables. A hypothesis predicts a relationship among variables.

Variables should be operationally defined. An *operational definition* assigns meaning to the variable by specifying the activities necessary to measure or manipulate the variable.

Independent variables are manipulated (actually or statistically) by the investigator in order to *measure changes* in the *dependent variable* that occur as a result of the manipulation. Independent variables influence dependent variables. *Assigned* independent variables are analogues of *active* independent variables; for assigned independent variables, the parameters of the variable are not actually manipulated, but sampling or statistical methods are used as "manipulative" factors. *Dependent variables* are *not* manipulated by the investigator, and they do not influence independent variables. They are expected to change when the independent variable changes, and they are measured to see if they do.

In most of the published research, the formulation of the problem is not presented as a specific section, and the reader must make some inferences about the nature of the problem from what is in the brief review of the literature presented as background material. The review will probably not reflect all the parameters of a problem, but the reader should be given enough information to identify the broad area of interest addressed by the investigator.

The *purpose* should be stated as such, and the variables in the research questions or hypotheses defined in terms of the measurement operations.

References

Babbie, E.R. The Practice of Social Research. 2d ed. Belmont, Calif: Wadsworth, 1979.

Brink, P.J., and M.J. Wood. Basic Steps in Planning Nursing Research, from Question to Proposal. 2d ed. Monterey, Calif: Wadsworth, 1983.

Cozby, P.C. Methods in Behavioral Research. 2d ed. Palo Alto, Calif: Mayfield, 1981.

Gay, L.R. Educational Research: Competencies for Analysis and Application. Columbus, Ohio: Merrill, 1976.

Kerlinger, F.N. Foundations of Behavioral Research. 2d ed. New York: Holt, Rinehart, & Winston, 1973.

Polit, D., and B. Hungler. Nursing Research: Principles and Methods. 2d ed. Philadelphia: J.B. Lippincott, 1983.

Wandelt, M.A. Guide for the Beginning Researcher. New York: Appleton-Century-Crofts, 1970.

Study Activities

1. Establish the relationship between problem, purpose, and research questions or hypotheses as these terms are used in the text.

2. Using the Alden formulation of the problem, state a study purpose. Identify three research questions that the study will answer.

3. Write a study purpose and research questions in which *quality of nursing care* is an independent variable; then write a study purpose and research questions in which *quality of nursing care* is a dependent variable.

4. List five active independent variables and five assigned independent variables that may be of importance in nursing.

5. Define *research question*; write five research questions. You may use the variables listed in study task 4.

6. Define *hypothesis*; write five hypotheses. You may use the research questions developed in study task 5.

7. Define *measured operational definition*. Write the measured operational definition of three nursing variables.

8. Define *experimental operational definition*. Indicate how this differs from a measured operational definition.

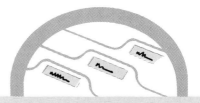

5

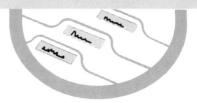

When you complete Chapter 5, you will be able to...

1. Explain the importance of the literature review.

2. List and define the steps in the library search.

3. Explain the activities of analyzing and organizing the literature.

4. Differentiate empirical material from theoretical material in a literature review.

ORGANIZING THE LITERATURE REVIEW

PURPOSE OF A LITERATURE REVIEW

The review of the literature related to the research problem begins with the effort to formulate the problem, and may even be the stimulus for the effort. It continues throughout the design of the study. A major question for the novice investigator is when to stop reading. This is also a major question for the experienced investigator, and you will see why this is so when you begin to learn all the good things a literature review provides.

A study should be based on the thinking and research that have preceded it; therefore, the investigator must know the relevant theory and previous research (Fox, 1969). Gay (1976, p. 24) defines a literature review as the "systematic identification, location, and analysis of documents containing information related to the research problem." This is pretty much what everyone else thinks it is. In reviewing the literature, the investigator finds out what has already been thought and done about the research problem, thus making the investigator a "subject matter expert" (Sweeney and Olivieri, 1981).

Knowing how other investigators addressed the variables of interest provides background for the current study and helps to refine the problem formulation and develop a rationale for the study by clarifying understanding and insight for the investigator.

Needless duplication can be prevented and suggestions as to what still needs to be done are found (Browne and Pallister, 1981; Cozby, 1981; Dempsey and Dempsey, 1981; Gay, 1976; Polit and Hungler, 1983; Treece and Treece, 1982). Furthermore, the review of the literature provides information about the research procedures and the instruments and measurements that have been useful in other studies (Fox, 1969; Gay, 1976).

The review will also help the investigator to interpret her findings, which can be considered in terms of whether they agree with what is already found in the literature—either the empirical studies or the theories. If the findings support the literature, she can consider the next problem; if they do not, she may suggest plausible reasons why they do not and consider whether the conflict is permanent or important (Dempsey and Dempsey, 1981; Gay, 1976). Fox (1969) suggests that it is always a good idea to review the literature in the context of the investigator's own study; he believes that the section on the literature should be written in anticipation of what will be needed in later sections of the study. One of the things that will be needed is some place to go with the findings. They cannot just sit there in splendid isolation; they must be lodged with the findings of earlier studies in some logical way.

If you are reading carefully, you will now be aware that the review of the literature is useful to the conceptual, the empirical, and the interpretive phases of the research process. Now, put yourself in the investigator's place and try to decide when to stop reading. Circumstances are likely to dictate the time, for instance, the dissertation is due, or the article was mailed yesterday to the journal editor. The review process itself, however, does give the investigator some hints about when to stop reading. She will notice that the information she is getting is repetitive and can be found in other studies. She will realize that the major studies in the field have been considered, and the reference sections of the articles she is reading include studies she has already considered.

LIBRARY TECHNIQUES

You will have assumed, correctly, that all this reading is taking place in a library, and frequently in more than one library. Nothing is more useful to the career of an investigator, or to the career of a student, than to become happy in a library. Learn the rules and the procedures. Browse; run your hands over the books, and read two or three just for fun. Smile at the librarian, and ask for help whether you need it or not. Librarians like to help you, and they know more than anybody else in the world. They can almost always recommend a book or a journal article that will be useful. Do not expect them to do your work, but do ask them to do *their* work, which will help you with yours. If you are serious about what you want to learn, they will be serious about it also (Gay, 1976; Polit and Hungler, 1983; Treece and Treece, 1982). Librarians are human, and they get tired and have headaches (just like nurses, after all), but they are a major resource for a serious reader. In any case, even if the librarian is cross, libraries, like gardens, are pleasant places to be; use them.

In the preceding and the following chapters, you are learning what it is an investigator *should* be doing so you have a standard of comparison when you read what was done. This chapter is a little different because the paired abilities of doing a literature search and writing a literature review are useful to students whether or not they are investigators. So, just for this one step in the research process, the intent is to help you learn to *do* it and not just to understand it. The guidelines for the investigator are equally useful to the student writing an essay or a report.

How does the investigator or the student use the library for a literature review, when she is ready to settle down to serious reading? Let us develop some guidelines with the help of several authors* who have written excellent chapters about how to do a review of the literature (Fox, 1969; Gay, 1976; Polit and Hungler, 1983). Fox says that the first phase of a literature review is to identify and read all the relevant published material. The second phase is trickier because that is when you write it all up, but let us deal with some guidelines for identifying and reading here.

1. The investigator should make a list of key words and phrases, which are obtained from the formulation of the problem, and use these to focus the literature search. An investigator who is interested in iatrogenic infection, for instance, should not be reading articles about patient satisfaction. Key words may be the names of variables. In a study of iatrogenic infection, hospital infection rates and handwashing techniques may be two key phrases.

2. As to sources of information, the place to start is in collections of indexes and professional abstracts. This is not the time to go drifting along the bookshelves, looking for appropriate titles. The card catalogue is indexed by subject (subject probably

*For a comprehensive understanding of both the process of a literature search and detailed guidelines for writing a literature review, consult the authors referenced (Fox, Gay, and Polit and Hungler). Their chapters on the subject are directed toward the development of a study, but the excellent advice they give should also be used by students reading for course work. Their texts are likely to be found in a campus library and are well worth consulting.

is the same as a key word or phrase). Also, there are computer bibliographies to which the librarian has access; by entering key words and phrases into a computer program, a printed list of appropriate articles can be obtained (Brink and Wood, 1983; Polit and Hungler, 1983). This is not as much fun as looking through the card catalogues and the journal indexes, but it is a lot faster. Because different libraries provide different resources, the librarian should be asked to help (Polit and Hungler, 1983). A further suggestion from Brink and Wood (1983) is to talk with people who know something about the topic, as part of the review activities.

3. It is not appropriate to try to include everything. The investigator should review the *related* literature, that is, the literature related to the current study. If the area is heavily researched, she looks at studies that are directly related to her study; if there is not much research around the problem, studies that are less directly related should be included (Fox, 1969; Gay, 1976; Polit and Hungler, 1983).

Fox (1969) believes that every reference should serve a specific, study-oriented purpose. However, be sure that all the information is obtained. In their discussion of the scope of the review, Polit and Hungler (1983) identify the kinds of information the investigator may need to acquire: facts, statistics, and findings; theory or interpretation; methods and procedures; opinions, beliefs, points of view; and anecdotes, clinical impressions, and narration of incidents and situations. Every investigator need not acquire all of this every time; this merely suggests the possibilities.

4. *Primary* sources must be sought. A primary source is the work of the person who developed the concept or the report of the study written by the person who did the study. It is the original work. It is not correct to depend on a reference to the original work made by another author. This is known as a secondary source. Secondary sources are often interpretive of the original work, so that an investigator should become accustomed to looking for the unadorned original (Fox, 1969; Gay, 1976).

How does the investigator begin to accumulate information? Abstracting the material involves locating, reviewing, summarizing, and classifying references (Gay, 1976). The investigator locates the article because it has one of her key words in the title. She reads the abstract, or the summary of the article, to see if it is one she wants to read. If it is, she scans the article, noting the main points. With regard to noting the main points, all the authors referenced in this chapter agree that there should be some consistent note-taking activity that comprehends all the necessary information, so the investigator will not have to look it all up again. They agree that putting the information on index cards is better than writing on the backs of old envelopes, and 4 x 6 is a useful size. The card should contain a complete bibliographical reference, including the library call number, in case the investigator forgets something and has to look again. A bibliographical reference to a journal consists of the author's name(s); the year of publication; the article title; the title, number, and volume of the journal; and the page numbers of the article. For books, the reference contains the author's name(s), the year of publication, the book title and edition, and the name and location of the publisher. For chapters in edited books, editors' names and chapter title and pages are added. This is not as involved as it sounds. The idea is to make access to the references easy; also, the complete citation will be required if the planned study is published. It is useful to follow a manual of style in the referencing so that the references are consistent in form.

After all that, the essential points covered are noted, as well as anything the reader thinks to say about the article at the time it is read. It is important to keep the points made by the writer separate from the comments made by the reader because later it is sometimes difficult to know which is which (Gay, 1976). A good way to do this is to use a lot of direct quotations in summarizing the main points of the article, remembering to include page numbers. It is a major mistake to postpone noting reader comments about the points in the article, since it will be difficult to recall them later, when they are needed for writing the literature review.

An investigator may become so attached to the joys of reading that there is reluctance to take on the joys of writing, but it must be done. When an imposing number of bibliographical references has been collected, it is time to begin making use of them.

ANALYZING AND ORGANIZING THE LITERATURE

Analyzing and organizing the literature means writing the literature review for the study. According to Gay (1976, pp. 34-35), the first step is to make an outline. Her guidelines are summarized below.

1. Make an outline, identifying the main topics in an appropriate order and developing subtopics as needed. The investigator must be prepared to rearrange and recast the outline if it does not agree with the references and to discard some references in the presence of a good outline that they do not fit.

2. Figure out which references go under which topics and

subtopics of the outline. See earlier remarks about discarding references, if necessary.

3. Take all the references for a given subtopic and analyze the differences between them; look also at the relationships. If several of the references report the same findings, write a summary statement, followed by all the authors' names. Do not write "Smith said A = B; Robinson said A = B; Johnson said A = B; Jones said A = B." Summarize: "There is general agreement that A = B (Johnson, 1969; Jones, 1971; Robinson, 1969; Smith, 1980)." Contradictory findings are analyzed and evaluated: "Although Smith says that A = B, Jones and Johnson report that A does not equal B. It is possible that the sample selection in the Smith study was subject to biases that had some impact on the findings." Note that *Smith* does not think she had a biased sample, but the investigator thinks so, and furthermore, she thinks that is why Smith's findings contradict the findings of Johnson and Jones. That is what the investigator tells *her* reader; she gives more than the information that Smith differs from the others; she suggests why that might be. This allows her reader to understand why she chose to follow the work of Johnson and Jones in her research, rather than the work of Smith, and indicates that she knows all the literature, not just the pieces with which she is in agreement. Chapter 6 contains a discussion of ways in which various authors classify design, and the paragraphs explaining why this book follows a certain classification system is one example of a short literature review.

4. The written review should flow in such a way that the least related material is presented first, with the most related material discussed last, just before the hypothesis or the statement of the purpose of the study. (Remember that *related* means related to the investigator's study.) The presentation of the literature should lead clearly and logically to a tentative, testable conclusion: the hypothesis. If the study does not test hypotheses, the review should lead to the statement of the purpose of the study and to the research questions.

5. The review should conclude with a brief summary of the literature and its implications. The summary should be detailed enough to show how the investigator got to the hypothesis or the research questions.

Fox (1969) says that the written review should include summaries of the major positions in the field and the major research findings that are relevant to the present study, plus the critical analysis by the investigator of the positions presented and the research. A review of the literature is always a *critical* review. Positions and findings are not simply reported without critical comment; they are organized into an original statement by the investigator, with the thought in mind that she needs a place to go with her findings when she gets them. It is not enough to write a series of book reports about the references. The points made by the authors must be compared and contrasted with one another and subjected to criticism by the person writing the literature review.

There are two kinds of material collected in the literature search: empirical material, that is, researchers' conclusions, the results of studies, and conceptual, or theoretical, material. Fox (1969, p. 114) differentiates them by defining the *research* literature (the empirical literature) as being the published reports of research studies that present data, and then assigning everything else to the conceptual literature. This literature will, therefore, include opinions, experiences, theory—any published material that does not report research findings. The conceptual literature is *data free*.

A review of literature for a research proposal must contain the literature of the empirical studies, the data-producing studies, and the literature of the theories and/or conceptual frameworks, the data-free papers, related to the variables of interest to the investigator. Information from both literatures must be present in the background material provided by the investigator to her reader.

A final note about writing a report of the study which may be useful to the student as a student, as well as a critical consumer of research.

The objective of scientific writing is clear communication, and it is the responsibility of the writer to provide clear communication. Writing styles differ, as well as levels of writing skills, and it is not the purpose of this book to teach writing skills. However, any college professor will support the need for students to acquire them. You will find a manual of style a useful reference for this purpose. There are many good ones to choose from, and their use will make your papers easier to write and easier to read. The Publication Manual of the American Psychological Association (APA) (1983), for instance, provides some comments useful to students writing papers.

In the section on Expression of Ideas (APA, 1983, pp. 31–36) there is terse and reasonably comprehensive advice as to the orderly presentation of ideas, smoothness and economy of expression, and precision and clarity in word choice. Strategies to improve writing style are presented briefly: writing from an outline; writing a first draft and re-reading it several days later; and asking a colleague to read the draft critically.

Remember that the investigator who has done a sound study is responsible for communicating the study process and results clearly. As a reader you have a right to expect an orderly presentation of ideas, smoothness and economy of expression, precision and clarity in word choice, correct grammar, and careful construction of sentences. The reader of *your* papers has a right to expect the same things.

SUMMARY

The investigator has two tasks with the literature. She must do a *library search* to identify and then read the literature that is relevant to her study, and she must *analyze* and *summarize* that literature for her reader.

The *study problem, purpose,* and *variables* must be reflected in the *written review,* and the *interpretation* of the study findings must be lodged there. No investigator works in isolation, and the works of others who are considering the same or similar variables must always be examined.

References

American Psychological Association: Publication Manual of the American Psychological Association. 3d ed. Washington, D.C.: American Psychological Association, 1983.

Brink, P.J., and M.J. Wood. Basic Steps in Planning Nursing Research, from Question to Proposal. 2d ed. Monterey, Calif: Wadsworth, 1983.

Browne, G.B., and R.M. Pallister. The research process: Literature review. In Y.M. Williamson, ed. Research Methodology and Its Application to Nursing, pp. 81-95. New York: John Wiley & Sons, 1981.

Cozby, P.C. Methods in Behavioral Research. 2d ed. Palo Alto, Calif: Mayfield, 1981.

Dempsey, P.A., and A.D. Dempsey. The Research Process in Nursing. Monterey, Calif: Wadsworth, 1981.

Fox, D.J. The Research Process in Education. New York: Holt, Rinehart & Winston, 1969.

Gay, L.R. Educational Research: Competencies for Analysis and Application. Columbus, Ohio: Merrill, 1976.

Polit, D., and B. Hungler. Nursing Research: Principles and Methods. 2d ed. Philadelphia: J.B. Lippincott, 1983.

Sweeney, M.A., and P. Olivieri. An Introduction to Nursing Research: Research Measurement and Computers in Nursing. Philadelphia: J. B. Lippincott, 1981.

Treece, E.W., and J.W. Treece, Jr. Elements of Research in Nursing. 3d ed. St. Louis: C.V. Mosby, 1982.

Study Activities

1. Indicate how the review of the literature may be useful to the investigator.

2. Indicate how the review of the literature may be useful to the student.

3. Write a short literature review, following steps 1 through 5 in the section Analyzing and Organizing the Literature. Use the reading required for any of your courses for this task.

4. Differentiate empirical material from theoretical material in the literature review developed in study task 3.

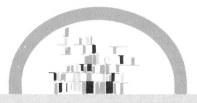

6

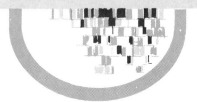

When you complete Chapter 6, you will be able to...

1. Describe the characteristics of exploratory design.

2. Describe the characteristics of descriptive design.

3. Differentiate experimental from nonexperimental design by
   a. Listing and defining the required properties of experimental design.
   b. Identifying difficulties in devising and implementing experimental design when the population is a population of human subjects.

4. Compare the three types of design (exploratory, descriptive, experimental) in terms of the kinds of evidence each provides.

5. Differentiate *ex post facto* design from experimental design.

TYPES OF DESIGN

A design is a strategy to get the information the investigator wants to have. There are two major aspects to developing a research design: the investigator must specify exactly what he wants to find out and he must determine the best way to do it. The point here is that if he is able fully and exactly to specify what he wants to find out, the best way to do it will fall into place fairly easily (Babbie, 1979, p. 83). Brink and Wood (1983, p. 89) define a design as a set of instructions to the investigator for gathering and analyzing data. It isolates variables of interest and indicates how to measure them accurately; it also indicates how the investigator gets rid of everything he does not want to measure, but that may affect what he does want to measure. The design is a blueprint for conducting the research. It contains plans for collecting, organizing, and analyzing the information. In general, the objects of a design are to give the investigator maximum control over the environment and the variables of the study and to make explicit how bias is avoided (Alexander, 1981; Selltiz, Jahoda, Deutsch, and Cook, 1966). Bias happens when data are collected in such a way that one answer to a research question is favored over another (Selltiz et al., 1966).

Mathematicians say that a properly formed question contains the answer within it. This may not always occur so clearly in social science, but it is useful to think along those lines. If there is a clearly formulated problem, an unambiguous statement of the purpose, and operational definitions of the variables, it is usually obvious enough what the data collection and data analysis plans should include.

For the pure in heart, there are only two basic approaches to research: experimental design and everything else, loosely described as nonexperimental design. Investigators who are seeking new knowledge in laboratories, where they exercise full control of environments and subjects, design experiments as a matter of course and may not even consider that anything else is scientific inquiry. Investigators who are studying variables in human populations may start in the laboratory, but sooner or later, they will be testing hypotheses in less well-controlled settings. We would all *like* to design experiments because there is no doubt that experimental design provides the best evidence for inferring that the research hypothesis is (or is not) supported. Sometimes we cannot do so.

Scientists like the *rigor* of experimental design, and research findings based in experimental design are *trustworthy* in a way that findings based in nonexperimental design are not. In the experiment, the investigator has been able to do certain things. Subjects have been randomly selected and randomly assigned to groups. Extraneous variance is controlled: this means that nothing but the independent variable is acting on the dependent variable. Most important, the investigator can manipulate the independent variable and measure the dependent variable. If he can do all this and describe what was done, he has experimental design and can rest comfortably with his findings, at least while he is in the laboratory, although problems may arise when the findings are tested in a less-controlled situation.

In a young science, though, the investigator may not be able to do experimental design. It is not that he does not know how; experimental design is, in a way, the easiest kind to write, since the rules about what you must do are clearly stated. But experiments demand certain kinds of control by the investigator. They also demand previous knowledge, and the investigator may not have this. The exploratory and descriptive work must be done before the experimental work; in older sciences, a great deal of such exploration and description has already been carried out; thus the investigator working in those sciences can afford to say that scientific inquiry equals experimental inquiry.

Nursing science is young. The theories are still developing, and empirical facts are not yet well organized. This will change as the theories are tested and the facts become organized under one or another theoretical framework. But it is naive to try to use experimental design just for the sake of having experimental design. The research design should be appropriate to the state of the knowledge about the variables.

Now, let two things be reiterated for clarity: the statements above do *not* suggest that nursing science does not support experimentation, nor that experiments are wrong. Many scientists in nursing are working with variables that are amenable to experimental design and are doing excellent experimental work that is advancing the science and the practice. But this is not the *only* kind of design appropriate to developing the science and the practice. Experimental design is undoubtedly the most useful for the advancement of nursing science. But in nursing, we are still exploring and describing, and the experiment is not useful for these tasks. Also, in nursing research, we are eventually dealing with human subjects: nothing can contaminate an experiment faster than a human subject. To summarize:

1. Nursing is a science and as such is advanced by testing hypotheses derived from nursing theory. This requires experimental design.

2. Experimental design provides the rigor necessary to trust in the findings.

3. Experimental design is possible only when the investigator has control of many elements: when subjects can be selected and assigned to groups in certain ways, when the independent variables can be manipulated and the dependent variables can be measured, and all other factors than the independent variable can be kept from having an impact on the dependent variable. If you think that all this sounds hard to do, you are right.

4. The discipline of nursing is concerned with people. When research subjects are people, the investigator begins to lose control of some of the elements of experimental design described in item 3.

5. When the depth of knowledge about the variables and the characteristics of the subjects allow it, experimental design is the best design—best because it provides the strongest evidence for accepting or rejecting hypotheses.

6. When experimental control is not possible, and the purpose of the study is to test hypotheses, the rigor of the experiment should be maintained as much as is possible. The necessary deviations from experimental rigor should be described and defended, and not simply taken for granted. The findings must be interpreted carefully, with the understanding that experimental control was not exerted.

Let us agree, however, that *scientific* inquiry is possible in other than experimental design, and discuss some of those designs. We will believe that a young science may require some research of a "pioneering character" in the presence of theory that may be either too general or too specific to provide clear guidance for empirical studies (Selltiz et al., 1966).

There are many ways to categorize research design; Gay (1976) discusses this in her classification of research by purpose and by method. In classification by purpose, she addresses the differences between basic research, to develop and refine theory, and applied research, the application of theory to resolve practice problems. She points out that the purpose of research and development (R&D) programs is to develop effective products for use, and the purpose of action research is the resolution of practice problems through the application of the scientific method. Such a classification is not informative concerning the components of the design, and she moves to a classification by method. She suggests that while all studies have certain common procedures (all the steps in the research process are carried out in some manner), each method is designed to answer a different kind of research question. She would place all studies in one of the following categories: the historical method, the descriptive method, the correlational method, the causal-comparative method, and the experimental method.

Fox (1969) uses a different classification by method and describes the historical approach, the survey approach and the experimental approach. Babbie (1979) does not classify; he identifies the purposes of research (exploration, description, explanation) and discusses sampling, measurement, and data collection techniques across kinds of studies in detail. He does devote separate chapters to the experimental method but does not attempt to classify research designs.

Wilson (1985) describes several typologies, including the basic-applied classification and a set of types of nursing studies classified according to purpose or method. Polit and Hungler (1983) identify experiments/quasi-experiments and nonexperimental approaches, and include survey and evaluation research, needs assessment, historical research, case studies, secondary analysis, and methodological research as additional types of research.

Beyond the agreement that there are experimental designs and nonexperimental designs, authors differ in how they classify the various kinds of research effort.

The design lays down the rules for the collection and analysis of the data, and it is apparent that major design differences will occur on the basis of the purpose of the research. The rules for data gathering are not the same for the investigator who is intent on exploring a concept about which little is known as they are for the investigator who is testing a theory-based causal hypothesis. Therefore, we will follow an older trail here and categorize designs on the basis of how they differ in purpose, that is, on the basis of the investigator's intent. The categories are not always distinguishable in practice, since any study may contain elements from any one of them, but we will distinguish them for discussion.

Selltiz et al. (1966) identify three types of design: exploratory design, descriptive design, and design to test causal hypotheses.

EXPLORATORY DESIGNS

Exploratory designs are created by the investigator in order to become familiar with the variables of interest and to gain insights into their relationships. Because the major emphasis is on the discovery of ideas and insights, the design must be flexible and amenable to change. If the investigator is in the field exploring variables and finds that variable A is not all that important after all, and that the relationship between B and C should be explored, the design must be alterable to allow him to do so.

According to Babbie (1979), exploratory designs are developed for three reasons: to satisfy curiosity, to test the feasibility of a more rigorous study, and to develop methods for a more rigorous study. Alexander (1981) sees such designs as useful in exploring areas of inquiry that do not have theoretical development. She believes that exploratory studies are designed to raise questions, not to provide answers. Brink and Wood (1983) say that in exploratory work, the variables are under the control of the situation and can only be observed as they happen.

Exploratory studies may have several purposes: to clarify the concepts of a problem or a methodology; to familiarize the investigator with a setting that he wants to use in a more structured study; to get information about the possible difficulties with a planned research activity; and to get an idea of the problems regarded as urgent by the people working in the field (Selltiz et al., 1966).

Those who would say that exploratory work is no doubt important, but only experimental work may be regarded as scientific are referred to Selltiz et al. (p. 52). They point out that "if experimental work is to have either theoretical or social value, it must be relevant to broader issues than those posed in the experiment. Such relevance can result only from adequate exploration of the dimensions of the problem with which the research is attempting to deal."

Even the most determined purist will admit that exploratory work must precede experimental work, and in sciences of greater intellectual maturity, this exploration has already occurred. In nursing, there is still a good part of it to do, and we must remember that the most rigorous methods in the later considerations of variables are useless if these considerations are based on early work that is irrelevant or incorrect (Selltiz et al., 1966).

In developing the parameters of a good exploratory design, Selltiz et al. (1966) suggest a good literature search, a survey of persons who have experience with the research problem, and the examination of insight-stimulating examples. They emphasize flexibility, since the investigator must change the research procedure to accommodate the data, as the accumulating information dictates a change in the direction of the approach.

Exploratory studies may be carried out under the rubric of scientific design and remain flexible as well as scientific. The investigator never simply goes into the setting to sit down and let the data happen. He has looked at the literature and talked with people in the setting. He knows a little about some of the variables and what the important relationships are likely to be, and he starts out with a study schedule that allows him to note the relationships. He is alert to the fact that he may need to start looking at another set of variables, using a different kind of observation. This attitude of alertness to the changing picture is of major importance in exploratory work. There is no point in trying to control, measure, and manipulate variables until there is some evidence suggesting which ones should be controlled, measured, and manipulated. The key word in exploratory design is *flexibility*.

DESCRIPTIVE DESIGNS

Descriptive designs are created by the investigator in order to make accurate statements about the characteristics of individuals, situations, or groups. The study may or may not contain hypotheses about the nature of these characteristics. Such designs may also be used to determine the frequency with which a variable occurs or is associated with another variable (Selltiz et al., 1966). A census is collected using a descriptive design; marketing surveys and political polls are descriptive approaches (Babbie, 1979).

There is a substantial difference of opinion about which research approaches should be classified as descriptive; there is some confusion with exploratory design (Alexander, 1981) and some use of a different terminology; for example, "correlational research" as described by Gay (1976) seems to be descriptive design. Alexander (1981) suggests that reference to the aim of the study will help the reader to distinguish the type of design. Some of these differences in conceptualization are described, since they are all in common use.

Descriptive studies, say Polit and Hungler, are "not concerned with relationships among variables. Their purpose is to observe, describe, and document aspects of a situation." They perceive that the "intent of such research is not to explain or understand the underlying causes of the variables of interest" (1983, p. 170). Dempsey and Dempsey (1981) believe that descriptive design (also called survey research by them) is present oriented—it describes what currently exists. Using this definition, they perceive the term as inaccurate, since description is involved in historical research, which describes the past, and experimental research, which describes what happens to B if A is manipulated. Gay (1976) also presents descriptive design as being concerned with testing hypotheses related to current status. Brink and Wood (1983) allow two categories of design: descriptive and experimental. They say that if you want to answer the question "what?" the design is descriptive. The choice of the design is made when the question is finalized. They combine exploratory and descriptive approaches and agree that in descriptive design, the investigator must know quite a lot about the variables before the study begins. For our purposes, we will look for those factors about which there is agreement, and we continue to find Selltiz et al. (1966) useful.

Descriptive studies describe the characteristics of a group: they identify relationships. They share, by whatever name they are known, two important characteristics.

1. The research question presupposes prior knowledge of the problem. The investigator must be able clearly to define *what* is to be measured, find ways to do it, and identify *who* is included in the population. That is, he needs a clear formulation of what and who are to be measured, and a technique to do so (Selltiz et al., 1966). Many epidemiological studies might be included in this research approach. We are always interested in the proportion of persons with certain health characteristics and in being able to predict the occurrence of these characteristics as they may be associated with demographic variables: the association of age of mothers with the occurrence of birth defects in infants, for instance, or age of mothers with the number of out-of-wedlock pregnancies.

2. The descriptive design is *not* flexible. The aim of the study is to obtain complete and accurate information, so the investigator must protect, in the design, against the bias inherent in flexibility. The time for investigator judgment calls about the importance of a variable is pretty much past in descriptive design. The key word in descriptive design is *accuracy*.

TESTS OF CAUSAL HYPOTHESES (EXPERIMENTAL DESIGNS)

To understand why everyone would rather design experiments than anything else, we need to talk a little about causal relationships: experimental design is needed in order to make inferences of causation, and although experiments may be designed merely to test association, a major purpose of experimental design is to test causal hypotheses. An inference of causation happens when you believe that A causes B, or has some influence on B, in certain specified conditions.

A hypothesis of a causal relationship says that a particular characteristic or occurrence in one variable, let us say variable X, is one of the factors that determines a characteristic or occurrence of another variable, usually known as variable Y (Selltiz et al., 1966). In the human inquiry kind of thinking about causality, a single event may be considered always to lead to another single event. If the investigator washes his car (event X), it rains (event Y). Obviously, the cause of rain in his area is car washing. Scientists are merely human, but their techniques of inquiry are not, and they conceptualize a causal relationship a little differently. They look for a *multiplicity* of determining conditions, which will make the occurrence of a given event *probable*; that is, they look for the *necessary* and *sufficient conditions* for an event. A necessary condition is present if X must occur in order that Y will occur. For instance, in order for chemical dependency to happen, prior experience with some form of drug must have happened. Prior experience (variable X) is a necessary condition for addiction (variable Y). A sufficient condition is present if X is always followed by Y: destruction of the optic nerve (variable X) is always followed by blindness (variable Y) (Selltiz et al., pp. 80-81).

Note that necessary and sufficient are not the same thing. Drug use is a necessary condition to addiction, but it is not a sufficient condition, since many people who experiment with drugs do not become chemically dependent. Variable X is necessary, but it is not enough. On the other hand, destruction of the optic nerve, while sufficient to cause blindness, is not necessary. There are other causes of blindness, so that variable Y can occur in the absence of variable X.

This concept of "determining conditions" is extremely important, and scientists are likely to speak of *conditional* rather than *causal* hypotheses.

In order to test a causal hypothesis, that is, to find out if X is a condition for Y, the investigator predicts that it is: he makes the hypothesis that "Variable X is a necessary condition for the occurrence of Variable Y." Then he designs an experiment to see if things happen that way, to accumulate evidence that X is related to Y in the way predicted.

There are three kinds of evidence required in order to infer that X is a condition for Y: concomitant variation, an appropriate time order for the appearance of the variables, and evidence that eliminates other possibly causal factors (Selltiz et al., 1966). This is why the investigator goes to the trouble to design an experiment, to accumulate such evidence in the most efficient and accurate way possible.

How does the evidence look? Evidence of concomitant variation is evidence of the extent to which X and Y vary together. Evidence of the time order of X and Y shows that X always happens first.

The X-Y occurrence may be simultaneous by the investigator's measure. Also, the relationship may be symmetrical, with each term in the relationship being both a cause and an effect of the other term. For instance, the higher the rank of a person in a group, the more likely he is to conform to group norms. On the other hand, the more he conforms to the norms, the more likely he is to attain high rank. Such simultaneous and symmetrical relationships may occur, but for our purposes, let us not be complex. We like the independent variable to precede the dependent variable. An elementary discussion stresses that one event cannot be considered the cause of another if it occurs *after* the other event (Selltiz et al., 1966). Therefore evidence of the time order of the two events is necessary for the inference of causality. If X happens after Y happens, X has not caused Y.

The third kind of evidence required, evidence eliminating other factors that *may* be causal, means that the investigator, in some way in his design, rules out the effect of all the other independent variables (X2, X3, X4, X5, etc.) that could possibly have any impact on Y.

Properties of Experimental Designs

The purpose of experimental design is to examine the effect of the independent variable (X) on the dependent variable (Y) in such a manner as to allow unambiguous interpretation of the results (Babbie, 1979; Cozby, 1981). In order for a design to be considered experimental, it must exhibit three properties: manipulation of the independent variable, control of variance, and randomization.

Manipulation of the Independent Variable. This means that the investigator does something, or causes something to happen to the subjects, and the something is different in the groups to which the subjects have been assigned. If the research purpose is to study the effect of reinforcement on behavior, one group of subjects may be rewarded and one group of subjects not rewarded for the same behavior. Reward is the operational definition of reinforcement, variable X. Then performance (variable Y) is measured, thereby providing evidence of whether concomitant variation has occurred: lots of reward in X, lots of performance in Y.

Control of Variance. This is a major function of experimental design, and indeed Kerlinger (1973, p. 306) says that the main technical function of research design is to control variance. Now, variance is a statistical term, and we will not deal with it here, but let us take what Kerlinger has to say about variance and move it to a less complex, nonmathematical level. Control of variance in an experiment means several things.

1. The investigator is able to maximize the difference between the experimental and the control groups. He can manipulate the independent variable so that the "experimental conditions" are as different as possible. In the reinforcement study, in the reward group, there are lots and lots of rewards: in the nonreward group, there is no reward. Reinforcement treatment A (lots of reward) is as different from reinforcement treatment B (no reward) as is possible.
2. The investigator is able to get rid of random fluctuation of the scores, a fluctuation that is not due to differences on the variable in the subjects. This variability is not predictable or systematic. It is not due to any bias on the part of the investigator. Errors of measurement contribute to fluctuation in scores, and one way to control error

variance is through establishing the reliability of the measure, the accuracy of the scores. The less error variance, the better.

3. The investigator in some way minimizes, or nullifies, or isolates, or rules out, or somehow gets rid of, all other possible independent variables than the ones being studied (Kerlinger, 1973, p. 309). He "controls" extraneous variables by putting together the study so that their impact on the dependent variable is nullified, or at least identified. There are three ways to do this: through elimination of the variables; through randomization (assigning subjects to groups in a manner that gives every subject an equal chance at any group); and through building the variables into the design.

   a. A variable can be eliminated as an independent variable by choosing subjects who are *homogeneous* on that variable. For example, if an investigator wants to look at the impact of reward on performance, how would he control for the impact of gender on performance, if his control principle was homogeneity on the variable? Right! He would sample only from a population of females. Or, of course, from a population of males.

   b. If, however, he was controlling the variable gender by means of *randomization*, he would sample from a mixed population and assign the subjects to the reward and nonreward groups in such a way that men and women had equal chances of being assigned to either group. This has the further virtue of controlling possibly competing variables that he did not know were there.

   c. The third method of controlling extraneous variables is to *build them into the design*. If the investigator thought that gender was making a difference, he might sample from a mixed population and randomly assign subjects to four groups: high reward, men; high reward, women; no reward, men; no reward, women. He would have four sets of scores (two reward sets, two nonreward sets) instead of two, and he would measure the effect of gender on performance in the presence of both levels of his reinforcement variable.

There is a word to help us remember the three factors in the concept of control: *maxmincon*. The researcher *maximizes* the difference of interest to the investigator in the experimental groups, *minimizes* differences owing to error, and *controls* differences owing to extraneous variables (Kerlinger, 1973, p. 307).

Randomization. The third property of experimental design requires that the investigator be able to assign subjects to the experimental or control groups on a random basis. The word *random* keeps coming up before you have read the definition. For right now, let *random* equal *by chance*. Random assignment means that each subject has an equal chance of being put in any of the treatment groups. The assumption is that if this is done, the differences in the groups will be due to the manipulation of the independent variable, not to different characteristics in subjects that the investigator has not measured and may not know about (Kerlinger, 1973). Such individual differences in subjects are considered to be "equated across groups"; for example, the reward group will have as many intelligent, assertive, high-achieving females as the nonreward group.

Obviously, the key word for experimental design is *control*.

Experiments may be categorized as either field experiments or laboratory experiments: both must exhibit the three properties described, and the distinction is based on the setting of the research. Field experiments occur in an existing situation: laboratory experiments occur in an artificial setting, contrived for the experiment by the investigator. In the laboratory, the investigator has total control of the environment, which makes it easier to design an experiment. However, the findings may not match what is found in a less artificial environment. Field experiments are shaky as to investigator control, but the realism is important (Polit and Hungler, 1983).

Such designs may be considered quasi-experiments, that is, designs that lack randomization or the control group component of experimental design. These designs are created to maintain as much experimental rigor as is possible in situations that are not entirely under the control of the investigator.

EX POST FACTO DESIGNS: A QUASI-EXPERIMENTAL APPROACH

One type of quasi-experimental approach common in health-related research is the *ex post facto* design. This is research in which the independent variable(s) has already occurred, and the investigator starts with the observation of a dependent variable(s) and examines various *possible* independent variables for their effect on the dependent variable.

We have seen that in experimental design, the investigator predicts from a controlled X to a measured Y: in *ex post facto* design, the Y is observed and a retrospective search for X occurs (Kerlinger, 1964). For example, in an experiment, an investigator predicts that in the presence of a certain chemical tar (variable X), skin cancer (variable Y) will occur. He paints the skins of a sample of laboratory rats with the chemical, controlling for extraneous variables such as kind of rats, age of rats, environment of rats, and waits. At a specified time, he counts the cancerous skin lesions. He has predicted from a controlled X to a measured Y, in an experimental design.

Another investigator is interested in the large number of cases of lung cancer, identified in morbidity and mortality statistics, and begins to see that the incidence appears greater in certain groups, for instance, groups who also report themselves to be heavy smokers. This investigator finds cases of lung cancer, variable Y, the *dependent* variable, and looks for plausible causes, variable X, the *independent* variable, among a multiplicity of possible causes (variable X1, variable X2, variable X3,...variable Xn, other possible *independent* variables). He studies each of these X variables in retrospect for their possible relation to, or effect on, Y. He has an *ex post facto* design.

The two major differences between *ex post facto* and experimental design are the control of the independent variable and the ability to assign subjects to groups in a random fashion. Inability to manipulate the independent variable(s) and self-selection of subjects into groups are important weaknesses in *ex post facto* design. Anytime there is group membership on the basis of a variable, self-selection is involved. The crux of the matter is that when assignment is not random, there is a loophole for the admission of other variables. When subjects are put in groups on the basis of one variable (e.g., cigarette smoking), it is possible that other variable(s) (e.g., genetic inheritance and anxiety) correlated with the X variable (cigarette smoking) may be the real basis of the association between X (cigarette smoking) and Y (lung cancer). Maybe people with certain gene structures who are anxious are also more likely to be heavy smokers, but they are more likely to contract lung cancer because of the gene structure and the anxiety, not because they are heavy smokers.

Well, we know how these studies came out, and the laboratory experiments with animals, which were *not ex post facto* suggest that the inference about the relationship between smoking and cancer is the correct one. The fact remains that it is dangerous to infer that X causes Y using only the evidence from *ex post facto* design.

Obviously, *ex post facto* design has some limitations: the lack of ability to manipulate independent variables, the inability to randomize, and the risk of improper interpretation of the findings. However, the investigator may try to move such designs toward rigor by testing alternative hypotheses, predicting and testing relationships between all other plausible Xs and lung cancer (Kerlinger, 1964), and this was done in the smoking studies.

Some of the more important variables in clinical nursing are not manipulable, and true experimentation is not always possible. Controlled inquiry by way of retrospective studies is an important strategy for the nursing investigator. The critical reader, however, must recognize the limitations of such designs and understand that the evidence of causality provided by the investigator using such designs must be interpreted with some care.

Note, however, that no matter what kind of design is involved, inappropriate interpretation may occur. An investigator who ignores faults in the design components and assigns meaning to his findings as though there were no design compromises misleads himself and his readers. Findings are only as sound as the design that provides the data, and no design is perfect. Whether the investigator is providing evidence of causality, or simply of relationships among variables, the limitations of the design in providing the evidence should be considered. However, when the investigator can predict from a controlled X to a measured Y—that is, when he has experimental design—he may assume that he has evidence at a satisfactory level of probability. Kerlinger (1964, p. 622) says that evidence at satisfactory levels of probability is sufficient for scientific progress.

SUMMARY

This chapter is general in nature; it tells you about a set of standard designs and what they may require from the investigator, but it does not say how they are developed. You need to know how designs may be classified so that you will know what kinds of control the investigator *should* have exerted. If you recognize that the investigator thinks he has an experiment, you will be alert as to how he controlled for extraneous variables and whether he manipulated the independent variable to your satisfaction. However, if the study is exploratory, you will understand that random selection of subjects is not a design requirement.

Research designs are classified here by the purpose of the investigator as *exploratory designs, descriptive designs*, and *designs to test causal hypotheses*. Designs to test causal hypotheses are *experimental designs*.

When the investigator has *little knowledge* of the concepts and variables of interest and is concerned with the *development of ideas and insights*, he creates an *exploratory design* that is *flexible* and amenable to change.

If he wants to make *accurate* statements about the *characteristics of a group*, to *identify relationships*, he creates a *descriptive design*. Descriptive designs are not flexible.

If he wants to *test causal hypotheses*, he must design an experiment. In an experimental design, the investigator must be able to *manipulate the independent variable, control variance*, and *assign subjects to groups on a random basis*. He predicts from a controlled X (the independent variable) to a measured Y (the dependent variable).

When it is not possible to design an experiment, *quasi-experimental designs*, which lack either the random or the control group component of experimental design, may be used. *Ex post facto design* is an example of quasi-experimental design that is commonly used in health-related research. In *ex post facto* design, the investigator studies a variety of possible independent variables for their possible effect on a dependent variable that has already occurred.

References

Alexander, C.S. Types of research design. In Y.M. Williamson, ed. Research Methodology and Its Application to Nursing, pp. 113-144. New York: John Wiley & Sons, 1981.

Babbie, E.R. The Practice of Social Research. 2d ed. Belmont, Calif.: Wadsworth, 1979.

Brink, P.J., and M.J. Wood. Basic Steps in Planning Nursing Research, from Question to Proposal. 2d ed. Monterey, Calif.: Wadsworth, 1983.

Cozby, P.C. Methods in Behavioral Research. 2d ed. Palo Alto, Calif.: Mayfield, 1981.

Dempsey, P.A., and A.D. Dempsey. The Research Process in Nursing. Monterey, Calif.: Wadsworth, 1981.

Fox, D.J. The Research Process in Education. New York: Holt, Rinehart & Winston, 1969.

Gay, L.R. Educational Research: Competencies for Analysis and Application. Columbus, Ohio: Merrill, 1976.

Kerlinger, F.N. Foundations of Behavioral Research. New York: Holt, Rinehart & Winston, 1964.

Kerlinger, F.N. Foundations of Behavioral Research. 2d ed. New York: Holt, Rinehart & Winston, 1973.

Polit, D., and B. Hungler. Nursing Research: Principles and Methods. 2d ed. Philadelphia: J.B. Lippincott, 1983.

Selltiz, C., M. Jahoda, M. Deutsch, and S.W. Cook. Research Methods in Social Relations. New York: Holt, Rinehart & Winston, 1966.

Wilson, H.S. Research in Nursing. Menlo Park Calif.: Addison-Wesley, 1985.

Study Activities

1. Indicate which type of design provides the most trustworthy findings and why.

2. Describe the characteristics of the design required if the intent of the investigator is to gain insight into relationships.

3. Describe the characteristics of the design required if the intent of the investigator is to make accurate statements about the characteristics of individuals, situations, or groups.

4. Describe the characteristics of the design required to test causal hypotheses.

5. List the kinds of evidence required in order to infer that X is a condition for Y. Define each term in the list.

6. State how *ex post facto* design differs from experimental design.

7. Differentiate *necessary* conditions from *sufficient* conditions. Give an example of each.

8. Define *maxmincon*.

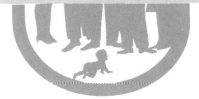

7

When you complete Chapter 7, you will be able to...

1. Differentiate populations from samples by
    a. Identifying the characteristics of a population.
    b. Identifying the characteristics of a sample.
    c. Explaining the differences in the characteristics.

2. Differentiate random samples from nonrandom samples by
    a. Listing and defining random sample techniques.
    b. Listing and defining nonrandom sample techniques.
    c. Explaining the major differences in the two kinds of selection techniques.
    d. Explaining the advantages and disadvantages in the use of either technique.

3. Differentiate random selection from random assignment.

POPULATIONS AND SAMPLES

POPULATIONS

Because nursing is a science of interaction, nursing research is usually concerned with populations of persons. Even when the populations studied do not consist of people (researchers in nursing may study cells under a microscope, or blood chemistries, or sheep uteri, or personnel forms, or other kinds of populations), the intent of the researcher is usually to be able eventually to say something about people and their responses to a health-care system.

We are dealing in this book with populations and samples of human beings. Identification of populations of interest and selection of samples from these populations must include consideration of the complexity of the organisms studied and the complexity of the researchers studying the organisms. The number and the complexity of the variables in any human interaction and the complexity of the systems in which humans interact have an impact on the design. The fact of consciousness (unlike cells observed under a microscope, patients observed during treatment know they are observed and respond to the fact of observation) and the existence of human rights are also factors in the investigator's strategy.

People do not have to be subjects in a research design if they prefer not to do so, and furthermore, they may change their minds at any time during the study and opt out of further cooperation with the investigator. This freedom constitutes a giant step for mankind, but it can be devastating to a research design. All these factors may have some impact on the study findings, and the investigator may or may not know what that impact is. Careful identification and description of the population and appropriate sample selection techniques may allow the investigator a reasonable level of comfort in making statements about a population on the basis of the findings in the sample, despite the factors mentioned earlier.

When investigators talk about *populations*, they mean those groups (of people or characteristics or atoms or microorganisms or stars) that they want to be able to say something about, the group in which they are interested. Now, almost any population is too large or too spread out for the investigator to study the entire group directly. There are usually many elements in a population; to look at each one would take too long and be too costly. Also, every element is not likely to be immediately accessible to the investigator, and by the time the element is accessible, the characteristics being studied may have changed. Therefore, the investigator does not study the entire population directly; instead, a small part is selected, that is, a sample. A sample is a portion of a population which is assumed to stand for, to *represent*, the entire group. In human inquiry, as well as in scientific inquiry, knowledge is based on samples. We inform ourselves about a few members of a group and make inferences about the whole group on the basis of what we know about a few members. Before we can talk about samples and how they are selected, a few definitions that are related to populations must be considered.

There is only a reasonable degree of agreement about the language used to define populations. Smith (1981) tells us about a general universe, which he says is an abstract theoretical population to which the researcher wants to generalize her findings. This is a hypothetical group, which may extend into the past and into the future. It is impossible to study that group directly, although it is the group that we want to say something about. Fox (1969) defines universe a little less comprehensively and says that it consists of all possible respondents or measures of a certain kind. He says that a population is the portion of the universe to which the researcher has access; Smith (1981) calls this a working universe, the universe from which the researcher will select her sample. Others define populations as consisting of all the cases meeting a designated set of criteria, as the people, things, or events of interest to the researcher (Babbie, 1979; Dempsey and Dempsey, 1981; Giovannetti, 1981; Polit and Hungler, 1983). For our purposes, we will be satisfied with populations and try not to think about hypothetical universes. Babbie (1979) finds the term useless; we will follow his lead and concentrate on real, definable groups, or populations. Although a population should represent its universe, in terms of application of the findings, if the investigator describes the population correctly, findings can apply to the population, even if not to the universe. What follows is a set of definitions related to populations. They are listed in descending order of size.

Universe: all possible respondents or measures of a certain kind (Fox, 1969); the theoretical and hypothetical aggregation of all elements defined, wholly unspecified as to time and place (Babbie, 1979). As you can see, universes tend to be large and a little amorphous.

Population: a theoretically specified aggregation of survey elements (Babbie, 1979); the entire aggregate of cases that meets a designated set of criteria (Polit and Hungler, 1983); the portion of the universe to which the researcher has access (Fox, 1969).

Target population: all the cases that meet a designated set of criteria (Giovannetti, 1981); the entire specified aggregate of cases for whom the investigator wants to generalize (Polit and Hungler, 1983). As an example, all cases meeting a designated criterion could be all nurses who are members of the American Nurses' Association.

Population strata: a population contained within another population (Giovannetti, 1981). For instance, in a population of hospitalized patients, all the male patients constitute one stratum and all the female patients constitute another stratum.

Population element: a single member of the population (Giovannetti, 1981).

In the definitions used by various authors, a population is the group that the researcher is interested in saying something about, and the group must be defined. Gay (1976) gives us a useful last word about populations. She says that a defined population must have at least one characteristic that differentiates it from all other groups. She also points out that the group the investigator would really like to get is probably not available, and therefore, the definition of the population must be realistic, rather than idealistic. She tells us that the first step in sampling is defining the population.

Let us look at an example of a population and some sampling activities. Imagine that you are the investigator who is interested in taste, and to do your study, you need to be able to give a taste score to a cherry pie. You consider the pie to consist of a population of taste atoms. How do you sample from this population?

Well, you do not eat the entire pie at one sitting; that is, you do not directly observe all the population elements. Even if you could do so without damaging your gastrointestinal tract beyond repair, by the time you finished, your taste buds would be so overwhelmed that they would shut down. The first bite would not have the same taste characteristics as the last bite, under a condition of satiety, so which information from the taste buds would you record? Is the score for the population (remember, all the taste atoms in the pie are the population) the score you give to the first bite, or the score you give to the last bite? Observing the entire population of taste atoms does not look to be a good idea.

However, if you eat one piece a day for a week, the variable of interest to you (the taste score) will change as the population (all the taste atoms) ages. What can you do? Well, you can assume that the taste atoms in the first piece you eat (the first sample) are just like the taste atoms in the rest of the pie, and you say that the pie is good because the piece is good; that is, you assign to the population the same score you gave the sample because you assume that the sample (the piece) represents the population (the whole pie).

If you were not sure that the first piece was representative, you could serve a piece to each of six raters (take six samples from the population, instead of only one), and let the taste score for the pie be the average of the six sample scores. This way, you do examine all the atoms (you use up all the possible samples for the population), but you have a new problem. You have to consider that maybe some raters do not like cherry pie, and this biases their scores. If the taste scores given their samples by two of the raters are low, does that say something about the taste characteristics of the population (all the taste atoms in the pie)? Or does it say something about some characteristic of your raters that may be contaminating your research? For this sample design to work, you have to be able to assume that the raters are alike; it might be better to let the first sample represent the pie.

It is obvious that even for the small population contained in one pie, that is, a population that can be accessed in its entirety, there are difficulties, and it gets worse.

What if the population is defined as all the Smith Bakery cherry pies ever baked or to be baked? What if we consider a universe of Smith Bakery cherry pies? Obviously, all these taste atoms are not accessible. What can you do? Well, you can identify a target population—maybe all the Smith Bakery cherry pies baked this week. You can select a daily sample and get taste scores for each sample. You could average the seven scores, and spend some time explaining that there is no reason to believe that the creation of the pies in the week you studied them differs in any meaningful way from the creation of pies all through the year. The thing is, you would like your taste score to be a Smith Bakery cherry pie score, not a Smith Bakery cherry pie score for the week of the investigation. You do not really care about the sample, that is, the selection from the pies baked in one week; you want to say something about the population of all Smith Bakery cherry pies. You want to *generalize* the sample findings to the population.

In order to do this, you must sample the Smith Bakery cherry pies in a proper manner, following some rules for the *selection* of the sample. The way you select the population elements into the sample allows you to generalize the sample findings to a population, or does not allow you to do so. Strictly speaking, you may only generalize sample findings to the population—that is, say that the sample does indeed *represent* the population—if you have selected the sample in a certain way and have what is called a probability sample, a random sample.

SAMPLES

Generally, sampling of any kind is considered to be the process of selecting a few elements from a population; these elements are expected to stand for all the elements in the population, on the characteristics of interest to the investigator. Always keep in mind that the investigator samples only to say something about a population.

Why sample at all? Why not just get the information from *all* the elements of a population, that is, do a census? The matters of cost and convenience were mentioned earlier—populations are usually large, and it is neither inexpensive nor convenient to observe or measure all the elements in most populations. Further, sampling may provide a more accurate picture than will measuring all the population elements, since it is easier to control sampling than it is to control a census (Giovannetti, 1981). A large survey, using interviewers, in which the entire population was interviewed, would necessitate training and maintaining an enormous staff, who would be difficult to supervise. It would also take a long time to get to everyone. Proper follow-up procedures would be difficult, and the time delay might affect the data. Giovannetti also points out that sometimes a sample *must* be used, for instance, in measuring blood levels; measuring blood hemoglobin on the entire population of red blood cells in an individual's vascular system would almost surely result in a lethal anemia, no matter what the laboratory findings were. It is also necessary to sample to measure knowledge, since no test can be comprehensive of all the knowledge about a concept.

The question in social science is not whether to sample, but how to do it in such a way that accurate conclusions about the many may be reached by studying a few (Babbie, 1979). How to sample resolves itself into who or what to observe, and how many observations to make. Who or what is observed is dictated in the main by the purpose of the study, the focus of the research. The investigator selects the set of observations that will provide the desired information about the variables of the study.

How many depends to a great extent on the homogeneity of the population. If all population elements are equal to one another, sampling one element will be enough. Physical scientists need not list all the carbon molecules and select a random sample to study; any old carbon molecule will do. Equally, physicians get the necessary information about blood levels from whichever 5 ml of blood happens to be drawn up in the syringe. Social scientists, faced with the heterogeneity of human subjects, require more controlled procedures; probability sampling is the efficient way to select a sample that will represent the variations in the population (Babbie, 1979). In a probability sample, the probability of inclusion in the sample can be specified for each population element, and no element is assured of inclusion in or exclusion from the sample.

Another problem is posed by human populations; human subjects have civil rights and may choose not to be in the sample, or to drop out at any time. It is worth remembering that even a probability sample of human subjects is (or should be—it is unethical not to give them the option) a probability sample of a population of volunteers. Because we do not usually know how the volunteers differ from the nonvolunteers, there is sometimes a question about the actual identity of the human population to which the sample findings are generalized.

The sample never represents a human population perfectly. In a probability sample, however, neither the researcher nor the subject can bias the selection. Also, a probability selection allows an estimate of the accuracy, the representativeness, of the sample; the investigator knows how likely she is to be wrong.

PROBABILITY SAMPLING TECHNIQUES

This section contains a set of definitions of the kinds of selection techniques in common use to get probability samples from human populations. Remember, a sample is a *probability* sample because of the way it is selected; it is the selection *process* that is random and bias free (Fox, 1969). The investigator goes to the trouble of setting up a random selection process (i.e., to do probability sampling) because she wants to say that the sample is representative of the population.

In such a sample, the probability of inclusion in the sample can be specified for each population element; usually each element has an equal probability of selection, but the requirement is that the probability of inclusion is known (Dempsey and Dempsey, 1981); no element should be assured of inclusion, 100 per cent probability of selection, or exclusion, 0 per cent probability of selection (Smith, 1981).

Before examining the kinds of random samples most commonly used in studies addressing health variables, let us look at the definition of two terms used in sampling: sampling element and sampling frame. A *sampling element* is a single member of a population (Giovannetti, 1981), and you have seen that definition before, in the section on populations. The *sampling frame* is the list of sampling elements from which the sample is selected. If a sample of patients is selected from a hospital registry, the registry is the sampling frame (Babbie, 1979; Giovannetti, 1981). Looking back to the definitions in the section on populations, you will discover that a sampling frame resembles a target population, and a sampling element and a population element are not dissimilar.

Simple Random Sample. In a simple random sample, each population element has an equal probability of being selected (Dempsey and Dempsey, 1981; Kerlinger, 1973), or the investigator can specify for every element in the target population the probability of its being included in the sample (Giovannetti, 1981). In order to select a simple random sample from a population, it is necessary to list all the population elements. If the sampling frame (the target population) is defined as all the patients in the Community Hospital on the day the data are collected, then a random selection from the list of patients is possible, although there would be some question as to what universe is represented by such a target population. The simple random sample is the model of the equal probability of selection method, but frequently it is modified in use. A major modification is the systematic random sample.

Systematic Random Sample. The selection of sample elements by taking every kth name on a population list is systematic random sampling. The list itself should be randomly ordered, and every population element must have a known chance of inclusion (Dempsey and Dempsey, 1981); it is the selection of the first element from the first k elements, using a random procedure, and selection thereafter at k intervals (Giovannetti, 1981; Kerlinger, 1973). This is not as involved as it sounds, but you need to know what some of the terms mean. Giovannetti (1981) provides a clear example: The investigator wants to select a sample of 100 individuals from a population of 1,000 individuals. The selection interval (known as k) is obtained by dividing the desired sample size (100) into the population size (1,000); the quotient is 10, which means that the selection interval (k) is 10; the investigator will select every 10th individual (every kth individual) until 100 are selected. The first individual is randomly selected from the first k individuals, that is, from the first 10 individuals on the list. How can this random selection occur? Well, the investigator could close her eyes and select a card from a deck; say that she chooses one of the 8s. The 8th individual on the list is chosen, and every 10th individual after that. This selects individuals numbered 8, 18, 28, 38, ... 998, into the sample of 100 individuals. Now that you understand the meaning of k, you may ask what is a randomly ordered list? It is one in which the place of each population element on the list is dictated by chance; it is developed in order that the selection interval is not the same as some periodicity in the data (Babbie, 1979).

Giovannetti (1981) tells us that the listing order must be random with respect to the measurement of interest, to avoid the possibility that the selection interval and the data have the same cycle. If the example was a list of health maintenance organization members who are husbands and wives and who appear alternately on successive lines of the list, a systematic sample that has an even-numbered selection interval would consist of all males, or all females. To avoid this, a random list of numbers can be generated and the selection of numbers made from that list, so the selection interval would not cycle with any characteristics of the population.

The simple random sample and the systematic random sample represent alternative methods for selecting a sample from a population list.

Stratified Random Sample. The stratified random sample represents a modification of the sampling frame (Giovannetti, 1981). In this sample, the population is first divided into strata, for instance, men and women; registered nurses, licensed practical nurses, nursing assistants; freshmen, sophomores, juniors, and seniors. Then a simple random sample is selected from each stratum (Kerlinger, 1973). The sampling frame is not the list of the entire population, but a series of lists by the various strata within the population. A target population might still be all the patients in the hospital, but the list from which samples are selected would be stratified by gender, if an equal number of men and women is desired.

The purpose of stratification is to organize the target population into homogeneous groups, with the population elements in each group as alike one another as possible, thereby obtaining representation of diverse elements within the population (Giovannetti, 1981); to organize the population elements into homogeneous subsets, with heterogeneity between the subsets; and to select appropriate numbers of elements from each subset (Babbie, 1979). Fox (1969) says that a sample (he calls it an invited sample, that is, the elements of the population that are selected into the sample) must represent the population on the levels of the variable in two ways—all significant aspects of the variable must be in the sample and each aspect must be present in the same proportion in the sample as in the population. Stratification assures that all levels of the variable are in the sample; proportional selection provides samples that represent the size of the levels in the different population strata. In a proportional stratified sample, subjects are selected in proportion to their number within the population, thus assuring internal homogeneity and that all significant aspects are represented in the sample (Chein, 1966; Fox, 1969; Polit and Hungler, 1983). The selection of variables for stratification depends on the purpose of the study and the availability of the variables. Age and sex are available to measure and are related to a lot of other variables of interest to investigators (Giovannetti, 1981).

It is not necessary to have the same number of subjects in each stratum, and indeed, it may be better to have a sample that represents the population in size of strata. For instance, in a target population that consists of the members of a health agency, the personnel assortment is 70 per cent registered nurses, 20 per cent licensed practical nurses, and 10 per cent nursing assistants. In a study of patient care, the investigator may stratify on status and select 100 individuals in proportion to the size of the status stratum in the population—70 registered nurses, 20 licensed practical nurses, and 10 nursing assistants (Giovannetti, 1981).

Cluster Sample. When it is not possible, or not practical to compile a list of the individual elements of a target population, but a list of groups of population elements is possible, cluster sampling may be used. A cluster sampling technique may be used in large-scale studies when the population elements are scattered and not easily listed singly. A cluster consists of groups of population elements with the same characteristics (Dempsey and Dempsey, 1981). The population elements are chosen in groups, not as individuals. The National Census Survey, for example, uses cluster samples and considers households, rather than individuals, for interview, although the population element is the individual, not the household.

Probability sampling is desirable; such samples can represent populations, since the investigator can specify the probability of selection of each element within populations. These techniques inhibit both conscious and unconscious selection biases in investigators, and the magnitude of the sampling error, that is, the difference between the sample value and the value in the population, can be identified (Giovannetti, 1981). However, even probability samples are not perfect; one can still get a biased selection from a human population because of a differential participation of selected subjects, for example, all those nonvolunteers who are selected and refuse to participate (Giovannetti, 1981).

Also, probability sampling is almost always an expensive effort and may be inconvenient. Frequently, it is impossible, since the investigator must be able to list population elements, or at least groups of elements, and she must make the best of what can be done, which is frequently some form of nonprobability sampling.

NONPROBABILITY SAMPLING TECHNIQUES

A nonprobability sample has a major disadvantage—the probability of selection of a population element is unknown;

therefore, there is no assurance that every element has a chance of being selected. Under these conditions, the investigator does not know if the sample represents a population, and in a study in which the investigator wants to generalize to a population, this is indeed a drawback.

Sometimes it is appropriate to use nonprobability, rather than probability, selection techniques, for instance, in an exploratory study, when the intent is to gain insights into the variables, or when the study focus requires subjects with some experience and competence. Further, the researcher may prefer to expend scarce resources on some other step in the research process rather than obtain a representative—and expensive—sample and, in any case, may be more interested in finding relationships among variables than in generalization (Cozby, 1981). In a realistic mode, Chein (1966) notes that a difference in probability and nonprobability sampling may only be on paper, since the plan for selection may not be properly executed. And sometimes there is no reasonable alternative to the nonprobability sample.

There are three common types of nonprobability samples: accidental samples, quota samples, and purposive samples.

Accidental Sample. In the accidental sample, the elements are simply conveniently there to study. In fact, this type is also called a convenience sample. Smith (1981) calls it a haphazard sample.

Quota Sample. A quota sample is similar to an accidental sample, in that the elements are conveniently there to select, but a step is added to ensure the inclusion of diverse elements of the population (Giovannetti, 1981). Controls are established so the sample is not overloaded with subjects having certain characteristics (Dempsey and Dempsey, 1981). For instance, in a quota sample of 100 subjects selected from a population of patients in a psychiatric hospital, an investigator who is interested in comparing patients who have a diagnosis of reactive depression with patients who have a diagnosis of manic depression would select 50 patients with each diagnosis: if she wanted to look at the impact of gender on behavior, the sample would be 25 females with manic depressive disease and 25 females with reactive depression, and 25 males with manic depressive disease and 25 males with reactive depression. By establishing diagnosis and gender quotas, the investigator is sure of having the two levels of each variable represented in the sample.

Purposive Sample. The purposive sample involves establishing criteria for selection and then selecting according to the criteria (Dempsey and Dempsey, 1981). Cases to be included are handpicked for their experience or knowledge or some other characteristic of interest to the investigator (Giovannetti, 1981).

RANDOM ASSIGNMENT

Despite the usefulness of the nonprobability procedures described, the importance of some effort to randomize cannot be overstated. Randomization is the basis of the investigator's statement that the sample findings may be applied to the population.

Random assignment grows out of the principle of randomization, as does random selection. Kerlinger states the principle of randomization as follows: "Since, in a random procedure, every member of a population has an equal chance of being selected, members with certain distinguishing characteristics— male or female, high or low intelligence, Republican or Democrat, dogmatic or not dogmatic, and so on and on—will, if selected, probably be counterbalanced in the long run by the selection of other members of the population with the 'opposite' quantity or quality of the characteristic" (1973, p. 123). He goes on to point out that this is not a law of nature; it is only what most often happens when random procedures are used.

Several of those procedures have already been mentioned— the probability selection techniques. Another set of procedures is concerned with the random assignment of subjects to groups and of treatments to groups. These events are different from one another and from random selection. They are best explained in an example.

Say that the head nurse introduced in Chapter 4, Priscilla Mullins, wants to establish a minimum schedule of turning, coughing, and deep breathing for patients who have had a general anesthetic. She knows what the intervention is, that is, how to help patients to turn, cough, and deep breathe properly. She does not know how often she must ask her nurses to do it for it to be effective. Her target population consists of all the patients on the general surgery unit who have had a general anesthetic, who are there during the time of her study and agree to participate. She establishes three experimental protocols: turn, cough, and deep breathe every 30 minutes; turn, cough, and deep breathe every hour; and turn, cough, and deep breathe every 2 hours. The techniques of turning, coughing, and deep breathing are the same for all groups, and the activity lasts for 48 hours in all three groups. The only variation is in the frequency of the effort.

She establishes a nonprobability quota sample of 30 patients per group, and she names her Groups A, B, and C. The first thing she does is randomly assign treatments to groups. Remember, the experimental variable is the frequency of the action of turning, coughing, and deep breathing, and the variable has three levels: every 30 minutes, every 1 hour, and every 2 hours. Each of these levels is assigned to one of the groups. She writes each of the three intervals on a piece of paper and puts the papers in a hat: the first paper drawn out of the hat is the interval assigned to Group A, the second is the interval assigned to Group B, and the third is the interval assigned to Group C. She now has randomly assigned treatments to groups, and she finds that the subjects in Group A will do the exercise every 2 hours, the subjects in Group B every 30 minutes, and the subjects in Group C every 1 hour.

Now she must assign her subjects (the patients) to the groups in some random manner. There are many ways to do this. A simple technique would be to go to a list of random numbers, and choose 90 numbers between 1 and 90 inclusive. The first 30 numbers in the list will be assigned to Group A, the second set of 30 numbers will be assigned to Group B, and the third set of 30 numbers will be assigned to Group C. She will choose each number only once. She is now ready to admit subjects to her study. She will admit 90 patients, and they will not all be coming into the hospital at the same time.

The patients are assigned the numbers 1 through 90 in a chronological sequence; the first patient to be admitted after she starts her study will be assigned to the group to which the number 1 was assigned, the second patient to the group to which the number 2 was assigned, and so on. In this manner the patients are assigned to the treatment groups in a random fashion, before they are admitted to the unit. Thus she has random assignment of treatments to groups (by means of the hat trick) and random assignment of subjects to groups (by means of the list of random numbers). She does not have random selection, since she takes the subjects who meet her criterion (general anesthetic during surgery) who are admitted during the time she is collecting data and are willing to participate. She admits subjects to groups until she has 30 in each group: a nonprobability quota sample, with random assignment of treatments to groups and random assignment of subjects to groups.

In the best of all possible research worlds, the investigator has the ability to do both random selection and random assignment of subjects to groups and treatments to groups. Nursing research, on the whole, does not occur in the best of all possible research worlds, but random assignment is often possible when random selection is not.

SIZE

The simplest statement to make about the size of a sample is the larger, the better, and then add the immediate qualifying remark that after a certain size is reached, increasing the size does not help much (Fox, 1969; Gay, 1976; Giovannetti, 1981; Kerlinger, 1973). Giovannetti (1981) tells us that as the population increases in size, the sample size required for precision in estimation remains constant, and the absolute size of the sample is more important than sample size relative to the population size. She says that equal precision (she is talking about a probability sample, and precision is concerned with how close the sample value is to the population value) is found in the following samples: when the population is 2,000, and the sample is 200, which is 10 per cent of the population, and when the population is 100,000 and the sample is 200, which is 2 per cent of the population. She says that the factors influencing sample size include the degree of precision desired, the variability in the target population, risk specification (this is how willing to be wrong the investigator is), and the procedure selected. There are some mathematical formulae for estimating sample size in probability sampling, which amount to educated guesses; these are based on simple random sampling, one variable, and are limited in their treatment of cost (Giovannetti, 1981). Gay (1976) suggests that the size of the sample depends, to a great extent, on the kind of study planned. Her rule of thumb is: for a descriptive study, sample 10 per cent of the population (20 per cent for smaller populations); for correlational studies, include 30 subjects for each relationship analyzed; for causal-comparative and experimental studies, 15 subjects per group, and 30 is better. Dempsey and Dempsey (1981) like a 10 per cent minimum for descriptive studies and 15 subjects per group for experiments. We will remember that bigger is better, up to a point.

SUMMARY

The groups of interest in nursing research, the *populations*, are likely to be human beings with human rights. These rights may impinge on the research design. Selection of a portion of the population, the *sample*, must be done following certain rules; if the sample is expected to *represent* the population, selection must be such that every *population element* has an equal or a known chance of being included in the sample.

A *target population* consists of all the cases to whom the investigator wants to *generalize*, that is, apply, the sample findings. Several kinds of *probability* samples may be selected from this group. A *simple random sample* is one in which each population element has an equal or a known chance of being selected. In a *systematic random sample* the choice of the first sample subject from the population is random, with every *kth* subject selected after that. In a *stratified random sample*, the population is divided into strata (for instance, men and women, in a population of students) and a simple random sample is selected from each stratum.

It is not always possible, or useful, to select a *random* sample, a probability sample, from the population. Some forms of *non-probability* samples are *accidental* samples, in which the investigator studies subjects who are conveniently there to study; *quota* samples, in which subjects are conveniently there and stratified on relevant characteristics, and a certain number is chosen from each group (50 men and 50 women, in a student population); and *purposive* samples, in which the investigator establishes criteria for selection and selects only subjects with those criteria (10 registered nurses who have experience in intensive care units).

Although nonprobability samples provide useful information, they have a major drawback, in that the investigator cannot apply the sample findings to the population from which the subjects were selected. However, *random assignment* of subjects to groups may be used, even when random selection is not possible, thus allowing the investigator to make careful generalizations to the population.

References

Babbie, E.R. The Practice of Social Research. 2d ed. Belmont, Calif.: Wadsworth, 1979.

Chein, I. An introduction to sampling. In C. Selltiz, M. Jahoda, M. Deutsch, and S.W. Cook, eds. Research Methods in Social Relations, pp. 509-545. New York: Holt, Rinehart, and Winston, 1966.

Cozby, P.C. Methods in Behavioral Research. 2d ed. Palo Alto, Calif.: Mayfield, 1981.

Dempsey, P.A., and A.D. Dempsey. The Research Process in Nursing. Monterey, Calif.: Wadsworth, 1981.

Fox, D.J. The Research Process in Education. New York: Holt, Rinehart, and Winston, 1969.

Gay, L.R. Educational Research: Competencies for Analysis and Application. Columbus, Ohio: Merrill, 1976.

Giovannetti, P. Sampling techniques. In Y.M. Williamson, ed. Research Methodology and Its Application to Nursing, pp. 169-190. New York: John Wiley & Sons, 1981.

Kerlinger, F.N. Foundations of Behavioral Research. 2d ed. New York: Holt, Rinehart, and Winston, 1973.

Polit, D., and B. Hungler. Nursing Research: Principles and Methods. 2d ed. Philadelphia: J.B. Lippincott, 1983.

Smith, H.W. Strategies of Social Research. 2d ed. Englewood Cliffs, N.J.: Prentice-Hall, 1981.

Study Activities

1. Differentiate populations and samples.

2. Discuss the inherent difficulties in selecting a sample from a human population, which are not present in sample selection in inanimate populations.

3. The purpose of a study is to determine if there is a relationship between level of education of the nurses, type of delivery of care,

and patient satisfaction with care, in oncology patients. Identify the target population and an appropriate sample selection technique. Identify the sample.

4. Assume that you have 1,000 charts in the files and that you want to select 100 of them to examine for the quality assurance protocol. Indicate which sample selection technique you would use and defend the choice.

5. Compare the characteristics of probability samples with the characteristics of nonprobability samples, and indicate the advantages of each selection technique.

6. Indicate how the principle of randomization may operate when random selection of the sample from the population is not possible.

7. Describe a research situation in which accidental sampling with random assignment of subjects to groups is used.

8. Defend the proposition that a small sample may provide the same precision in estimation as a large sample.

8

When you complete Chapter 8, you will be able to...

1. List and define the various data collection techniques.

2. Indicate the characteristics that make observation a scientific tool.

3. Compare the advantages and disadvantages of *observation* with the advantages and disadvantages of *self-report* to collect study information.

4. Identify the advantages and disadvantages of the use of available data as a data collection technique.

5. Compare the two self-report techniques by
   a. Indicating the advantages and disadvantages of each technique.
   b. Indicating the appropriate question format for each technique.
   c. Indicating the advantages and disadvantages of question formats.

DATA COLLECTION
TECHNIQUES

Before we begin to look at the various data-collection techniques, it may be useful to consider the word *data*. It has been used several times in the preceding chapters, usually with the general meaning of "information gathered for a research purpose." Although that is a perfectly good way to describe the meaning of the word, information all by itself is not really "data." Information becomes data when the investigator does something with it.

Suppose John Alden, the staff nurse who formulated such a fine problem in Chapter 4, obtains the following information about the patients and the nurses on his oncology unit. Mr. A is terminal, and Nurse H spends 20 minutes a day with him, Nurse I spends 15 minutes a day with him, Nurse J spends 6 minutes a day with him, and Nurse K never goes near him. Mr. B is going home in good shape, and Nurse H spends 80 minutes a day with him, Nurse I 60 minutes a day, Nurse J 26 minutes a day, and Nurse K never goes near him. Ms. C is getting better rapidly after her mastectomy, and Nurse H spends 60 minutes a day with her, Nurse I 75 minutes, Nurse J 32 minutes, and Nurse K never goes near her. Ms. D is expected to die during this hospitalization, and Nurse H spends 25 minutes a day with her, Nurse I spends 35 minutes, Nurse J 22 minutes, and Nurse K never goes near her.

John Alden now has some information about his patients and about his colleagues; for one thing, he has information that leads him to believe that Nurse K should probably get into another line of work, but he does not have *data* yet. He must organize the information in some way appropriate to his study focus. He might develop a data sheet that looks like this.

NURSE MINUTES SPENT

PATIENT PROGNOSIS

	H	I	J	K
A: Terminal	20	15	6	0
B: Not Terminal	80	60	26	0
C: Not Terminal	60	75	32	0
D: Terminal	25	35	22	0

Now he begins to have data; he has juxtaposed the values of the variables for each of the subjects in the two groups. It is just information until he puts it together in some way dictated by the framework of the study. Babbie (1973) suggests that scientists do not collect data; they create it by asking questions. The questions determine the answers. John Alden has created data about the impact of the medical prognosis of patients on nurses' behavior by obtaining information about the prognoses of a set of patients and defining nurses' behavior in terms of the amount of time spent with patients by nurses. Different data would have been created if behavior was defined as initiating interaction, rather than as time spent. Babbie is making a pitch for operational definitions, for thinking in terms of making useful measurements, not indicating some ultimate meaning. The investigator creates the data set by establishing the categories of response to his questions.

For our purposes, data collection involves getting the information that is useful to the study, and organizing it in some way. The step of data collection shares a characteristic with several of the other steps in the research process: different authors define the step in different terms (Brink and Wood, 1983; Gay, 1976; Polit and Hungler, 1983; Treece and Treece, 1982). In this book, we will usually follow Selltiz, Jahoda, Deutsch, and Cook (1966); they identify three data-collection methods: observational methods, questionnaires and interviews, and projective and other indirect methods. We will move away from them a little, however, and identify data collection in terms of where the information comes from: *observation*, by the investigator; *self-report*, by the subjects; and the *use of available data*, that is, the use of information already collected by someone else. Projective techniques (that is, the interpretation by the investigator of subjects' responses to stimuli considered capable of generating a variety of responses) use all of those sources, as does placing individuals on some form of rating scales. We will organize data-collection techniques in terms of how the information is obtained: observation by the investigator, report by the subject, or the use of information obtained by information gatherers who were not concerned with the study.

OBSERVATION

Observation is like sampling in that it is an integral part of human inquiry. The observer is a watchbird, watching and noting the behaviors of people or animals or watching and recording events of interest. The watchbird collects information about what is occurring and records the information. Records may be in narrative form, including everything observed, with no effort to process the information, or the observer may have a *schedule*, a form with categories to which behavior or other events may be assigned. For example, an observer may simply note that little Johnny smacked little Mary, that he took her doll, that he offered her a bite of his cookie, and that he smiled. Or, if the investigator is using a formal observation schedule, he may put two check marks in the aggression category, one check mark in the friendly category, and one check mark in the cheerful category.

Observation methods are useful when the study intent is the description and understanding of *behavior as it occurs*. It is not effective if the investigator wants to describe cognitive or affective activities or values, perceptions, beliefs, or feelings. Future plans, past behaviors, and private behaviors cannot be studied by observation.

Observation is also like sampling in that the rules change when observation becomes a technique of scientific inquiry. It is a scientific technique when it has the following characteristics (Selltiz et al., 1966).

1. It serves a formulated research purpose.
2. It is planned systematically.
3. It is recorded systematically and related to a set of general propositions (the investigator has to be more than merely curious).
4. It is subject to controls for reliability and validity.

The observer, the information collector, is considered a part of the instrument, since he is also an information processor. Frequently, a major task of the observer is to assign the behavior being observed to some category (Kerlinger, 1973). In the example given earlier, the observer may have to decide whether little Johnny's behavior when he smacks little Mary is hostile or merely assertive and then check the appropriate category.

Observation may serve several research purposes: the technique may be used in exploratory studies to gain insights; it may be used to provide supplementary information that will help to interpret findings generated using other data-collection techniques; it is a primary technique in descriptive studies designed to describe situations and in experimental studies designed to test causal hypotheses.

It is a technique that may be used in either field or laboratory settings. The observation procedures may vary from a flexible set of observations guided only by the purpose of the study to a formal schedule with detailed response categories. Participation in the situation by the observer may also vary from none to a kind of participant observation, which is, in effect, membership in the group being observed. The degree of structure and the degree of observer participation vary with the purposes of the study (Selltiz et al., 1966).

Whatever the purpose of the study or the amount of structure of the observation schedule, the use of observation as a data-collection device requires that the investigator consider four questions: What should be observed? How should it be recorded? How can the accuracy of the observations be assured? and What relationship exists between the observer and the subjects being observed, and how is the relationship established? (Selltiz et al., 1966).

The question of the content of the observations is a problem in the selection of which behaviors to watch. In exploratory studies, in which the investigator does not know which variables are important, the degree of structure in the observation schedule is minimal. As understanding of the situation evolves, the content of the observation is likely to change, that is, the focus of observation shifts. The observer takes cues as to what should be observed from the events (Selltiz et al., 1966). In descriptive and experimental designs, the investigator knows which behaviors to observe and how they will be analyzed; therefore, he can set up well-defined procedures for assigning the observations to categories. Remember, in these designs, the observations must be related to some general propositions. There is not freedom of choice as to what is observed, and the observer will make an effort *not* to see those things that are irrelevant to the response categories. The instrument dictates to the observer both what is observed and how and where the information is recorded. Smacking people is always recorded in the hostile box, and snatching toys is always recorded in the assertive box. The observations are structured by the schedule.

How observations are recorded boils down to two questions: When should an observer make notes, and how should they be kept? The answer to "when" is on the spot and during the event, to avoid error because of a poor memory or because of poor selection among memories. If immediate recording will disturb the subjects, or if constant note taking interferes with the quality of the observations, key words should be noted, imperceptibly if possible, and the observer should remove himself from the situation whenever he can to make more detailed notes. However the immediate observations are recorded on site, the complete account should be written as soon as possible. The investigator should provide some information on these points in the research report. The more structured the observation, the less problem with recording, since some form of checklist, rating scale, or other categorized document will be used (Selltiz et al., 1966), and these may be used immediately and inconspicuously.

Considerations of reliability and validity are addressed by improving the accuracy of the observations and indicating the relationship of the observer to the situation. Accuracy is improved by using two or more observers, preferably with different cultural backgrounds and experience, for the same event. In these days of high technology, a sample of behaviors may be filmed to check the observer notes. Clear definitions of the kinds of behavior that are to be observed and how the behaviors are to be categorized are required. Error occurs in the presence of observer fatigue or because of the personal values of the observer, either of which may dictate how information is processed before category assignments are made. Careful and reiterated training of observers is the major defense against poor reliability owing to observer error (Selltiz et al., 1966), and the investigator should discuss this in the report of the research.

Although people become used to the presence of a watcher in a surprisingly short time, the presence of the observer may change the behavior of the subjects being observed. Techniques to nullify this must be developed before the data collection occurs. Full agreement by subjects to the observations and a neutral, nonthreatening watcher allow subjects to get used to being watched and continue in their normal ways. However, Kerlinger's admonition should be kept in mind by both the investigator and the reader of the report. He (1973) says that the major difficulty with observation as a data-collection technique is the observer, who must make the observation (get the information) and make the inferences necessary to process it (assign the behavior to the proper category), preferably without causing any changes in the behaviors being observed.

There are three advantages to using observation as a data-collection technique: behavior can be recorded as it occurs; the technique is independent of the subjects' *ability* to report; and the technique is independent of the subjects' *willingness* to report.

Observation is desirable in any study in which distortion of recall will affect the data. Further, observation provides information about behavior that subjects take for granted, and therefore are unable to report. Information can be collected from nonverbal subjects (infants, comatose patients, animals) using observation techniques. Subjects who refuse a verbal report because they do not want to give it the time, or do not want to be singled out, can be observed, although this is not as easy as it used to be, since it is usually necessary to get their permission for the observations. Observations may provide more accurate data than do self-reports in the presence of an unwilling or deceitful subject, since it is more difficult to alter behavior than it is to alter a memory for a self-report. Of course, unwilling subjects are not supposed to be subjects at all.

There are some disadvantages to observation. The investigator cannot predict or cause some spontaneous events. If he is interested in studying behavior in a disaster, he must wait for a fire or flood, or some equally appalling event, to occur and take himself there to observe the behaviors. Even regular events are not always observable. If the investigator is studying leadership behavior in a series of head nurse meetings, he may find that meetings are canceled or that permission to observe is canceled if the head nurses want to discuss hospital policies in private. The events he wants to study may be limited in duration, so that he cannot get all the information he needs. And finally, although letting it all hang out seems to be the policy today, there are still some behaviors that may be reportable but are not accessible to direct observation (for instance, sexual behavior, family crises, jury deliberations, consultations with physicians) (Selltiz et al., 1966).

SELF-REPORT

When collecting data by using the observation technique, the investigator obtains information by observing the subjects directly. In the self-report techniques (questionnaire, interview), information is solicited from the subjects (Gay, 1976).

The information consists of subjects' verbal or written reports about their experiences, perceptions, feelings, beliefs, and behaviors; to the extent that they have self-knowledge and are willing to share it, the investigator may obtain information not otherwise available. However, self-reports, by definition, consist of material that the subjects are both able and willing to report; there is some need to be able to estimate the validity of their reports. Accurate presentation of the facts might be embarrassing to a subject, so that he may embroider them a little. He may be reluctant, or indeed unable, to report his beliefs or feelings accurately (Selltiz et al., 1966). Given that the subject is both able and willing to report accurately, questionnaires and interviews can provide valuable information.

You know what a questionnaire and an interview are, but let us consider them as sources of information for a research study. In a questionnaire, the information obtained is limited to the written responses of the subjects to prearranged questions. In an interview, the subjects and the investigator are both present as the questions are answered. Therefore, even if the questions on the interview are prearranged as to wording and order, which they probably are not, there is a greater flexibility in the attempt to elicit information than there is with the questionnaire. Further, since the investigator is watching the subject respond, he can observe both the subject and the total situation, and he can estimate when he needs to rephrase a question and when the subject seems to be under some stress in replying to the questions. There are such things as telephone interviews, and certainly if the interviewer is not physically present with the subject, he is less able to make the estimations described. However, he can still move toward clarification of subject responses and reiteration of questions if the subject does not seem to comprehend, so the statement about greater flexibility stands.

In this section, we will consider these two types of conscious self-report, questionnaires and interviews, and compare them as to their usefulness and structure.

Questionnaires and interviews are both useful forms of data collection but for different reasons. Interviews are useful when the investigator wants to obtain information about issues that are complex or emotional or for probing sentiments, perceptions, or beliefs (Selltiz et al., 1966). They provide rich, difficult data. Questionnaires are limited to issues on which the subjects have clearly formulated views that can be simply expressed, and there is a general understanding that this is their best use (Selltiz et al., 1966). However, as will become evident later, with the use of certain kinds of questions, they can also generate rich, difficult data.

Both questionnaires and interviews may vary in form. Interview schedules may range from a standardized document in which the questions and the set of responses from which the subjects must choose are predetermined to an unstructured format in which neither the questions nor the response choices are predetermined by the investigator. The less structured format is more difficult to administer and is commonly used for intensive study of facets of the affective domain. Although the strength of the format is the flexibility it affords the investigator to probe for meaning in the responses, some effort must be made, even in the most flexible of situations, to keep subject replies specific and concrete, self-revealing, and spontaneous. The weakness of the technique is the lack of comparability of those same spontaneous responses and the consequent difficulty in analysis (Selltiz et al., 1966).

A final remark about this: Do not ever believe that the less structured interview is casual. Although it is used in an open kind of interaction, it is carefully planned, and the interviewer knows what he wants the subjects to talk about (Kerlinger, 1973).

Within the standardized format of the questionnaire, the amount of structure may vary by means of the type of questions asked. Two types of questions are used, and these are defined in terms of the kinds of responses they allow. In a *fixed-alternative*, or *closed*, question, the responses of the subjects are limited to the alternatives provided by the investigator. "Do you stay on your diet? Yes. No. Usually" is a fixed-alternative question. Another form is, "Why do you not stay on your diet? (1) weak willed, (2) like to be fat, (3) can't afford the protein, (4) don't believe it works." In both examples, the subject is required to choose one of the responses provided by the investigator.

An *open-ended* question permits free response from the subjects. An issue is raised, but the investigator does not structure the response in any way, although once the responses are obtained, he will certainly be required to assign them to some categories. In an open-ended format for the same two questions, the investigator would simply ask, "Do you stay on your diet? Why do you not stay on your diet?" and provide some white space on the form for the subject's responses.

In a standard format, the questions are presented in the same wording and same order to all the subjects, whether the questions are fixed-alternative or open-ended. When open-ended questions are used in a structured interview, the task of the interviewer is to encourage the subjects to talk freely, but to the point of interest to the investigator, and to record the replies. He may not raise new questions except to clarify the meaning of the responses, and these questions must be entirely nondirective (Selltiz et al., 1966).

There are advantages to the investigator in using fixed-alternative questions. They are simple to administer and inexpensive and easy to analyze. The answers are always usable in the analysis. Sometimes the alternative answers clarify the meaning of the question. If the subject does not understand "marital status" in a question about marital status, the responses labeled *Single, Married, Widowed, Divorced* indicate what the question means. Finally, the subject makes the judgment about which response to choose. Although he is limited to the responses provided, the investigator does not second-guess him in the analysis of the content, as happens with the responses to the open-ended questions.

There are some drawbacks, however, to using fixed-alternative questions. For one thing, they may force a statement of opinion from a subject who really has none. "Do you agree with Section 6 of the 1983 national budget? Yes or No." Most subjects will not have the faintest idea of what is in Section 6 of the 1983 budget, or even if there is a Section 6, but some will circle one of the responses just to be friendly.

Or there may not be a choice that corresponds to the opinion of the subject. Omission of possible alternate responses leads to bias, even if "other, please specify" is included as one of the choices, so unless the investigator is pretty certain that the alternate responses cover the range of possibilities, the fixed-alternative format probably should not be used.

The final drawback is that despite the same wording for all subjects, different subjects make different interpretations of the question, and the investigator can never know whether they do or not, or whether it makes any difference that they do.

Open-ended questions have their drawbacks too—nothing is perfect. They are difficult to analyze, since categories for analysis must be created and people trained to read the responses and code them into one of the categories. They are useful, however, when the study issues are complex and the relevant dimensions are not known to the investigator. If the study focus is the exploration of a process or the formulation of issues, open-ended questions are most useful.

Closed questions are efficient when the possible number of alternative replies is known, clear-cut, and limited in number. The closed question focuses the subject's attention on what is of interest to the investigator but does not allow him to provide information about his own formulation (Selltiz et al., 1966).

Most investigators use both question formats in the same instrument, choosing the question format that is most appropriate for the kinds of information desired and trying to maintain an adequate balance of formats to enhance the response rate. Few subjects want to write 50 essay responses, and if they are asked to do so, the questionnaire will go into the wastebasket, not the mailbox.

When interviews and questionnaires are compared in terms of the advantages and disadvantages of each, it is seen that questionnaires are less expensive and take less skill to administer. They can be mailed to a large number of subjects; thus it is possible to get more information from more people scattered over a wider geographic area than is possible with an interview technique. The subjects are more comfortable with assurances of anonymity, and there is less pressure for immediate response. The standardized nature of the instrument ensures uniformity in measurement, although not necessarily uniformity in meaning, since the meaning of the questions, even in standardized instruments, may be perceived in different ways by different subjects.

In semistructured interviews, *without* standardization of the question set, however, comparability is always an issue. On the other hand, interviews can be used with illiterate and very young subjects. They may yield a better response rate, since almost everyone will talk at length, even those subjects who do not want to write at length.

USE OF AVAILABLE DATA

Available data consist of recorded material that was not collected with the research purpose in mind (Treece and Treece, 1982). These documentary data are ready-made. The data were not collected specifically to provide information relevant to the interest of the investigator, but for administrative or legal reasons, or simply at the whim of a diarist or a newspaper editor.

Angell and Freedman (1965) categorize documentary material as *expressive documents* and *statistical data*. Expressive documents are such things as letters, diaries, accounts of small-group processes; statistical data include registration data, census data, and combinations of the two. The authors suggest that expressive documents are valuable in exploratory research, rather than in hypotheses testing, since randomization is a problem. They point out the impossibility of setting up a random sample from a universe of persons such that each member of the sample produces a spontaneous document for scientific purposes. Even if the sample is obtained and the subjects produce documents to order, they are not equally satisfactory for study purposes. Reliability of the interpretation of such data would appear to be in question, but these authors suggest that well-trained coders will agree to a satisfactory degree. The accuracy of the writer of the documents is always in question, as anyone knows who has done patient chart audits in an effort to identify the quality of nursing care on a unit.

Registration data consist of records made at the time an event occurs, to fulfill legal or administrative regulations attached to the event. This data set includes the registrations of vital events (births, deaths, marriages, divorces, morbidity) or education variables, of criminal activities (police records, parole records, court actions), of voting records, social security payments and benefits, automobile registration, military service, hospital records, and the records of activities of formal organizations. These data are useful to the scientist, for example, the epidemiologist, who wants to compare specific characteristics in different places at different times. They may be used to study relationships between variables relevant to a research problem, to select matched groups, and to select groups that differ on a characteristic being studied.

A census is a periodic collection of data about a population— any population, any period. The national census comes to mind as an example, but a disease census may be obtained in a population of children or a population of cities. The point is that the information, whatever it is, is collected at stated intervals from a population, not a sample.

The fundamental limitation to the use of documentary data is that they were not collected for the specific purpose of the research (Angell and Freedman, 1965). Therefore, they may be incomplete and may not easily fit the conceptual framework of the investigator, and usually, the investigator will not know the conditions under which the information was collected (Treece and Treece, 1982).

Advantages in the use of such data sets are that it is usually economical in time and effort for the investigator to use already extant information and sometimes the documents are the only source of information (Treece and Treece, 1982). Further, if the data were biased in some way while they were collected, at least they are not likely to be biased by the investigator in the direction of his hypotheses.

In evaluating such data for study use, the investigator must consider whether the recorder was motivated to secure or present accurate information. He must consider whether the regulations covering the record keeping may have changed, and he must know something of the definitions and contexts of the material in the documents that may affect his use of the data. Any information collected by persons other than the investigator is necessarily suspect; however, since it is unlikely in a complex study that the investigator will be gathering his own material, this difficulty is met in all data collection (Angell and Freedman, 1965).

Selltiz et al. (1966) add a further category of available data documents, *mass communications*. They assign literary productions, newspapers, magazines, motion pictures, radio and television programs to this general set. Some computer data bases may also be considered available data documents.

Any of the techniques of generating data have their strengths and weaknesses. The investigator who uses two methods of obtaining the same information is worthy of applause from his critical readers *if* the two methods have different weaknesses. If the responses of patients who are subjects are the same on the Satisfaction Scale (self-report technique) as they are on the hospital chart (nurses' observations), there is reason to believe in the accuracy of the information. Study findings are strengthened by using more than one method of acquiring information. Unfortunately, so are study expenses. Whatever the method of choice in data collection, the investigator should provide enough information about the technique that the reader may make some inferences about whether the choice is appropriate.

SUMMARY

Data-collection techniques are organized in terms of how the information is obtained: direct observation of the subject by the investigator, *observation technique*; response of the subject to investigator's questions, *self-report technique*; and the use of already extant information, *available data*, which was not gathered for the research, but for some other purpose.

Observation methods are useful when the investigator's intent is to describe and understand behavior as it occurs. These methods are independent of subjects' willingness and ability to report.

The *self-report methods* described are *questionnaire* and

interview techniques, in which information is solicited from the subjects. These techniques can elicit information not otherwise available to the investigator, but the subjects must be willing to share it. Format for the questionnaire or the interview may range from *standardized*, that is, questions and response sets from which the subject chooses are predetermined, to an entirely *unstructured* interview schedule, in which neither the questions nor the possible answers are predetermined.

Two kinds of questions are used in questionnaires and interviews: *fixed-alternative* questions, or *closed* questions, in which subjects must choose from responses provided by the investigator; and *open-ended* questions, which permit free response from subjects.

Available data consist of recorded material that was not collected specifically for the research study. The documents used may be *expressive*, for instance, diaries and letters, or *statistical*, for instance, registration data and census data. These data sets provide economy in time and effort for the investigator and are not amenable to bias in the direction of the study hypotheses. However, they may not easily fit the conceptual framework in which the study is based, and they are likely to be incomplete. Also, the conditions under which the information was collected are frequently not known by the investigator.

All the methods have some strengths and some weaknesses. In a good study, the investigator uses more than one method of collecting data, and the methods will have different strengths and weaknesses.

References

Angell, R.C., and R. Freedman. The use of documents, records, census materials and indices. In L. Festinger and D. Katz, eds. Research Methods in the Behavioral Sciences, pp. 300-326. New York: Holt, Rinehart & Winston, 1965.

Babbie, E.R. Survey Research Methods. Belmont, Calif.: Wadsworth, 1973.

Brink, P.J., and M.J. Wood. Basic Steps in Planning Nursing Research, from Question to Proposal. 2d ed. Monterey, Calif.: Wadsworth, 1983.

Gay, L.R. Educational Research: Competencies for Analysis and Application. Columbus, Ohio: Merrill, 1976.

Kerlinger, F.N. Foundations of Behavioral Research. 2d ed. New York: Holt, Rinehart & Winston, 1973.

Polit, D., and B. Hungler. Nursing Research: Principles and Methods. 2d ed. Philadelphia: J.B. Lippincott, 1983.

Selltiz, C., M. Jahoda, M. Deutsch, and S.W. Cook. Research Methods in Social Relations. New York: Holt, Rinehart & Winston, 1966.

Treece, E.W., and J.W. Treece, Jr. Elements of Research in Nursing. 3d ed. St. Louis: C.V. Mosby, 1982.

Study Activities

1. Differentiate *information* and *data*.

2. List the advantages of *observation* as a data-collection technique.

3. Compare *questionnaire* with *interview* as to the kinds of information each self-report technique is likely to generate.

4. Compare *questionnaire* with *interview* in terms of the advantages and disadvantages of each self-report technique.

5. Write a short questionnaire that will provide information to an investigator interested in patient satisfaction with care. For each item, indicate what the response will tell the investigator and why the question takes the form it does (fixed-alternative or open-ended).

6. Develop a set of research questions that could be answered using the technique of observation. Explain why observation is the best technique to use for these questions.

7. Discuss the advantages and disadvantages to the use of available data as a data-collection technique.

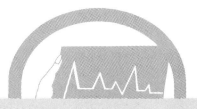

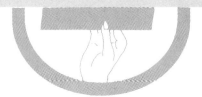

9

When you complete Chapter 9, you will be able to...

1. Differentiate the four levels of measurement.

2. Differentiate *reliability* and *validity* by
   a. Describing the kinds of reliability and indicating how coefficients may be obtained.
   b. Describing the kinds of validity and indicating how they may be established.
   c. Explaining the importance of the information concerning reliability and validity.

MEASUREMENT

You know what measurement is, and you are right: it is how much, or how many, or how big, or how long of anything. In a more technical mode, Siegel (1956) says that measurement is usually assigning numbers to observations in such a way that the numbers can be analyzed under certain rules.

LEVELS OF MEASUREMENT

Coombs (1965) tells us that the theory of measurement consists of a system of distinct theories, each corresponding to a *level* of measurement. The point for our purposes is that at each level of measurement, the data set must satisfy the assumptions of the theory for that level; if the assumptions are not met, it is not legal to measure the data at that level. This means that some levels of measurement are not appropriate for some data sets. There are four levels of measurement: the nominal level, the ordinal level, the interval level, and the ratio level.

Nominal Level or Classificatory Scale. In its simplest form, measurement consists of substituting symbols (usually numbers) for real phenomena. These symbols constitute a nominal scale (Coombs, 1965). Do you remember a variable called Gender? It has two attributes: Male and Female. All the responses or observations for that variable must be assigned to one of the attributes, and there must be an attribute for every response. This says that the attributes must be exhaustive (all the possible responses have an attribute to be placed in) and mutually exclusive (each response can be assigned to only one attribute).

The nurse completing a census report, who counts and records the number of males and the number of females on the unit, is using a nominal scale of classification. In nominal measurement, there is only classification by attribute. This is the lowest level of measurement.

About the only kind of measurement that can be carried out with nominal data is counting. One can count how many responses there are in each group and develop a *frequency distribution*, or calculate the percentage of women in the total sample, or the ratio of males to females.

The nominal level of measurement provides the least information to the investigator (Babbie, 1979; Kerlinger, 1973). Sometimes it is all she can get, and sometimes, for instance, in an exploratory study, it is all she wants.

Ordinal Level, or Ranking Scale. Frequently the objects measured are more than simply different from one another; they have more or less of the variable of interest (Coombs, 1965). Thus attributes may be rank ordered such that different attributes represent more or less of the variable. Order is inserted into the data from high to low. One familiar *rank order* is the letter grading system: A is greater than B; B is greater than C; C is greater than D; D is greater than F. F is not greater than anything. If the name of the variable is "knowledge of course content," then the understanding is that students who receive A know more course content than students who receive B or C; the Bs know more than the Cs, who know more than the Ds. The Ds probably know more than the Fs, but it is to be noted that a grade of F is *not* synonymous with knowing zero course content. There is no absolute zero in an ordinal scale. The nurse who assesses patients' condition and assigns every patient to one of the categories of critical, serious, fair, and good, is using a ranking scale.

The numerals assigned to ranked objects are called *rank values* and indicate *only* rank. They do not indicate absolute amounts, and they say nothing about the intervals between the numbers (Kerlinger, 1973).

Interval Level, or Interval Scale. Interval measures possess the characteristics of nominal and ordinal measures; that is, they are exhaustive, mutually exclusive, and have rank value. They also use equal distances between numbers, which are assumed to represent equal distances on the property being measured. The *intervals* can be added and subtracted.

Let us consider an interval measure that a nurse uses every day—a clinical thermometer. Farenheit or centigrade, it does not matter. The actual numerical value of each of the patients' temperatures is of interest and is recorded. The distance between the numbers on the scale (the thermometer is the scale) has meaning and is equal; that is, the distance between 97° and 99° is the same as the distance between 101° and 103°.

If you are looking at a weather thermometer rather than a clinical thermometer, the same thing holds. The distance between 80° F and 90° F is the same as the distance between 40° F and 50° F, but 80° is not twice as warm as 40°. Because the zero point on the scale is arbitrary, 0° F does not equal zero amount of the variable (heat). Nor does minus 30° mean 30° less heat than zero heat (Babbie, 1979).

In social science, there are techniques that develop the concept of "equal-appearing intervals," allowing the investigator to take advantage of certain powerful statistical manipulations that require at least interval measurement.

Ratio Level, or Ratio Scale. The strongest (this means the one that provides the most information) level of measurement is ratio measurement. Ratio measures have a "true zero," and in ratio measurement, 80 is twice 40. These measures have all the components of the lower levels, plus the true zero; a value of zero really means that there is none of the variable. All the arithmetic activities may be used at this level, and the numbers are assumed to indicate actual amounts of the property being measured (Kerlinger, 1973).

There are more variables at this level that are of interest to nursing than you might think. Age, medication dosage, weight, amount of formula taken, number of days hospitalized, amount of time spent teaching a patient are all ratio scales. Unfortunately, some of the most important nursing variables (nursing perform- ance and patient outcomes, for instance) generate measurement at lower levels. Fortunately, there are conventions and techniques that will help to move ordinal level data to interval level status. There are also good statistics for dealing with ordinal data.

Whatever the level of the data, the study findings cannot be trusted if the instruments used by the investigator do not provide scores that are both valid and reliable. These terms were defined in Chapter 2 as referring to whether the instrument provides the information that is desired, and whether it does so without fail. The questions are measurement questions, and a brief overview of how they are addressed follows.

RELIABILITY

Babbie (1979) says that reliability is a matter of whether a technique applied repeatedly to the same objects gives the same results every time. Gay (1976) agrees; she says reliability is the degree to which a test consistently measures whatever it meas- ures. Reliability is concerned with consistency, with dependabil- ity, with stability (Kerlinger, 1973). Please note that reliability is not necessarily concerned with accuracy (Babbie, 1979). You can set your scale back by 10 pounds, get on it daily, and get a *reliable* weight score; that is, if your weight does not change, the scale reading does not change. It is hardly an *accurate* reading of your weight, though, since it informs you consistently that you are 10 pounds lighter than you are.

Kerlinger (1973) does include accuracy in his discussion of reliability. He says that the question of reliability that is considered in elementary discussion of the subject is whether, when we measure the same object lots of times with the same or comparable instruments, we get the same or similar results. This considers reliability in terms of stability, dependability, and predictability.

However, he points out (1964) that there are two other questions that may be considered in the approach to reliability: Are the measures obtained the "true" measures of what is being measured? and How much random error is there in the measurement? The question about whether the measurement obtained is the "true" measure is a question about the accuracy of the instrument. Reliability can also be defined as the absence of errors of measurement in an instrument: the more error, the less reliability. Selltiz, Jahoda, Deutsch and Cook (1966) also suggest that an evaluation of the reliability of an instrument consists in determining how much variation in the values of the scores is due to inconsistencies in the measurement.

We will stay with the definitions used in elementary discussion of the subject (stability, dependability, predictability) and look at some methods used to estimate various kinds of reliability. When an investigator is providing you, the reader, with numerical estimates of the reliability and validity of the instruments used to collect and score the data, she must always indicate what *kinds* of reliability and validity are being estimated. Three kinds of reliability—internal consistency, stability, and equivalence—are considered below, along with how they may be established.

Internal Consistency. Estimates of the internal consistency of an instrument are concerned with whether all the items in the instrument are measuring the same thing. A teacher who wants to determine what a student knows about nursing diagnosis does not include questions about professional issues on the test. She may, however, include questions about physics if the nursing diagnoses framework she uses has a "related to" function: disorientation related to decreased oxygen in the blood, for instance. Internal consistency is estimated by determining how all the items on the instrument relate to the other items and to the total score (Gay, 1976).

If all the items measure the same thing, then the item scores should resemble one another and should resemble the total score in magnitude. A student who does not understand about nursing diagnosis on item 1 is not likely to do any better on item 2 or 6 or 8 if all the items measure the same content area.

Stability. Selltiz et al. (1966) say that stability is an estimate of the consistency of the measures on repeated applications. The coefficient of stability (the coefficient is the numerical estimate) indicates the degree to which scores are consistent over time. In order to obtain this estimate, the investigator administers the same instrument to the same group at different times. If the property being measured has remained stable, the scores on the instrument should not differ greatly at the two times (Gay, 1976).

Equivalence. The statement of equivalence is the statement of the extent to which *different investigators* using the same instruments to measure the same individual at the same time, or *different instruments* applied to the same individual at the same time, provide consistent results (Selltiz et al., 1966). The coefficient of equivalence is obtained by giving two forms of the same instrument to a group at the same time. The instruments purport to measure the same variables. Equivalent forms' reliability is established by computing the relationship between the scores obtained by administering two forms of the same instrument to the same subjects at the same time (Gay, 1976). This general statement includes a special kind of equivalence called *interrater reliability*, in which two investigators administer the same instrument to the same subject at the same time. Sometimes we must find out if the persons administering the instrument are "equivalent forms."

All this is important because if the instrument used to *measure* the variables is not dependable, the *relationship between the variables* cannot be established. Reliability is a necessary, but not a sufficient, condition for the instrument. Kerlinger (1973) says that reliability is like money; the lack of it is the real problem. It is also like money in that it is fairly easy to figure out how much you have; the reliability of the measure is easier to evaluate than the validity of the measure.

VALIDITY

Validity is the degree to which a test measures what it is supposed to measure. You never ask if an instrument is valid; you ask for what is it valid and for whom. The validity of a measurement can only be evaluated in terms of its purpose. An investigator must inquire into the nature and the meaning of her variables in order to estimate validity. The most common conceptualization is to ask whether the investigator is measuring what she thinks she is measuring. There is no one validity; an instrument is valid for the scientific or practical purposes of the investigator (Gay, 1976; Kerlinger, 1973).

Generally, the literature identifies content validity, construct validity, and two kinds of criterion-oriented validities: concurrent and predictive (Kerlinger, 1973; Gay, 1976; Selltiz et al., 1966).

Content Validity. Content validity, the extent to which an instrument measures an intended content area (Gay, 1976), is determined by expert judgment. Content experts know what should be included in the instrument, given its intended purpose. They compare this with what the investigator has actually included. This type of validity is composed of both *face validity* and *sampling validity*. Face validity is simply a question of whether the test content does indeed include the intended content area. Sampling validity is a question of how well the test content samples the total content area. For example, in a test designed to measure knowledge of nursing facts, there is good face validity if all the items deal with nursing; there is poor sampling validity if all the items deal with nursing of children.

Construct Validity. This type of validity indicates the degree to which a test measures an intended hypothetical construct. A construct is a nonobservable trait that explains behavior. In research, a construct must be defined operationally in terms of its indicators. The construct validity of an instrument is established by using the instrument to test hypotheses derived from the theory. If the hypotheses are supported, so is the theory **and** the construct validity of the instrument (Gay, 1976). This is double dipping at its best. Before you exclaim how easy it all is, be assured that it takes a good many replications of the same sort to establish the construct validity of an instrument. It all has to come out right more than once.

Concurrent Validity. Concurrent validity estimates the degree to which the scores on one instrument are related to the scores on another already established instrument, or to some other valid criterion available at the same time (Gay, 1976). If an investigator wants to establish the validity of a new anxiety test, she will give it to a set of subjects. She will then give them an already established anxiety test, the criterion test. If there is a high correlation between the scores, the assumption is made that the new instrument is a valid measure of anxiety. Another way to establish concurrent validity is to identify a group of people whom everyone agrees is a highly anxious group and another group whom everyone agrees is not anxious. If the measure can differentiate the groups, it may be considered a valid measure.

Predictive Validity. The degree to which a test will predict how an individual will do in some future situation is predictive validity. It is the degree to which an instrument is the predictor of some *future* criterion. The difference between predictive validity and concurrent validity is a time difference: concurrent validity predicts to some current criterion and predictive validity predicts to some future-based criterion. Both are criterion oriented. Kerlinger (1973) makes the point that for the criterion-oriented validities, *why* the instrument predicts is not important, only that it does. For construct validity, the investigator needs to know why.

Validity of any kind is concerned with the extent to which an empirical measure can adequately reflect the meaning of a concept. Babbie (1979) points out the tension in the relationship between reliability and validity. The specification of operational definitions of variables, which is done to ensure reliability, invariably leaves out the richness of meaning that is associated with the variable of interest. Anxiety is certainly more than a scale score, but it is the scale score that is reliable. There is always a question about the "real" meaning, the validity, of the scale score.

There is another way to look at validity, which must be mentioned here because you will see it discussed when you are reading research articles. Campbell and Stanley (1963) discuss validity in terms of the threats to validity and the kinds of designs that may control for those threats. They present a series of quasi-experimental and experimental designs for the consideration of the researcher and indicate for each one how it inhibits threats to internal validity and external validity. The question of internal validity is the question of whether differences in groups can be attributed to the experimental variable. The question of external validity is the question of when, or whether, the sample findings can be generalized to the population.

When you are ready to write proposals and move to an advanced research text, you will want to learn which designs control which threats to validity. This book gives you only the definition of the terms, so you will recognize the words and know their general meaning. It is the responsibility of the investigator to provide readers with comprehensive information concerning the reliability and the validity of the data-collection instruments. This information should include the level of measurement of the data.

SUMMARY

Data are considered to exist at various levels of measurement. Levels identified in the text are nominal level, ordinal level, interval level, and ratio level. In nominal level data, there is classification by attribute, and the measurement activity is essentially a counting activity. When data are at the ordinal level, it is possible to rank order on the basis of attributes of a variable. Numerals assigned to ranked objects indicate only rank and do not indicate absolute amounts. Interval level data use intervals between numbers, which are assumed to represent intervals in the data. If data are at the ratio level of measurement, intervals between numbers are used and a true zero is present.

The reliability and validity of the measurement tools must be established by the investigator. Reliability is concerned with the stability, dependability, and predictability of the measure.

Three types of reliability are considered in this book. These are *internal consistency*, which is concerned with the question of whether all the instrument items are measuring the same concepts; *stability*, which is an estimate of the consistency of the measures on repeated applications; and *equivalence*, the statement of the extent to which different investigators using the same instruments to measure the same subjects agree, or the extent to which different instruments applied to the same subjects at the same time provide consistent results.

Validity is concerned with whether a test measures what it is supposed to measure. *Content validity* is the extent to which an instrument measures an intended content area. *Construct validity* indicates the degree to which an instrument measures a hypothetical construct. *Concurrent validity* is an estimate of the degree to which scores on one instrument are related to scores on an already established instrument. *Predictive validity* is the degree to which a test will predict future behavior.

Another way to discuss validity is in terms of threats to *internal validity* and *external validity*. Internal validity is concerned with whether differences in groups can be attributed to the experimental variable; external validity is concerned with whether the sample findings are generalizable to the population.

References

Babbie, E.R. The Practice of Social Research. 2d ed. Belmont, Calif.: Wadsworth, 1979.

Campbell, D.T., and J.C. Stanley. Experimental and Quasi-experimental Designs for Research. Chicago: Rand McNally, 1963.

Coombs, C.H. Theory and methods of social measurement. In L. Festinger and D. Katz, eds. Research Methods in the Behavioral Sciences, pp. 471-535. New York: Holt, Rinehart & Winston, 1965.

Gay, L.R. Educational Research: Competencies for Analysis and Application. Columbus, Ohio: Merrill, 1976.

Kerlinger, F.N. Foundations of Behavioral Research. New York: Holt, Rinehart & Winston, 1964.

Kerlinger, F.N. Foundations of Behavioral Research, 2d ed. New York: Holt, Rinehart & Winston, 1973.

Selltiz, C., M. Jahoda, M. Deutsch, and S.W. Cook. Research Methods in Social Relations. New York: Holt, Rinehart & Winston, 1966.

Siegel, S. Nonparametric Statistics for the Behavioral Sciences. New York: McGraw-Hill, 1956.

Study Activities

1. Differentiate the four levels of measurement described in the text.

2. Differentiate *reliability* and *validity*.

3. The investigator has four raters making observations of the nursing care given in a clinical setting and has provided each of them with a standardized rating scale for nursing performance. Indicate what estimate(s) of reliability will be important here and why.

4. Describe the activities of an investigator who wanted to obtain estimates of equivalence and stability.

5. Compare *content validity* with *construct validity* in terms of what each kind of validity tells the investigator and how each kind of validity may be established.

6. Compare *concurrent validity* with *predictive validity* in terms of what each kind of validity tells the investigator and how each kind of validity may be established.

7. Define *internal validity* and *external validity*.

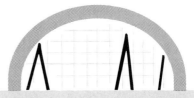

10

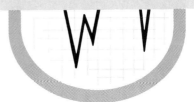

When you complete Chapter 10, you will be able to...

1. Differentiate *data analysis* and *data interpretation*.

2. List and define the rules for categorization.

3. Differentiate *descriptive statistics* from *inferential statistics*.

4. Describe how an investigator seeks a broad meaning of the findings.

5. Explain the relationship between data analysis and data interpretation.

DATA ANALYSIS AND INTERPRETATION

Now it is time for the investigator to move back to the armchair and sit and think some more. He spent a lot of time doing that in the conceptual phase of the research process. Maybe he moved to the library now and then, but the planning phase, the conceptual phase, generally can be carried out sitting down somewhere. The empirical phase requires a lot of activity in the real world to test the instruments for reliability and validity and to use them to collect information about the variables in the study. We can assume that the investigator continued to think, but he probably did not sit down much during this phase. Finally, though, the information is collected, and the investigator can return to the armchair to organize it and figure out what it all means.

Data analysis is part of the interpretive phase of the research process and consists of arranging all the information so that it tells something about the research question. It is mostly done sitting down, or maybe crawling about on the floor, trying to find the right stack of questionnaires. There is probably a computer operation somewhere, but the computer does not just chew up the questionnaires and spit out ordered data sets. The investigator has to do that and then hand-feed the computer with the ordered information. At any rate, he is no longer collecting data, but is organizing it.

That is what *data analysis* is: categorizing, ordering, manipulating, summarizing the data in the effort to obtain answers to the research questions (Kerlinger, 1973). It is to be contrasted with *interpretation*, also part of the interpretive phase, in which the investigator takes the results of the analysis and says what they mean. Data analysis provides the investigator with answers to the research questions: for example, the mean of Group 1 is greater than the mean of Group 2 at a significant level of probability; patients are more likely to express satisfaction on the primary nursing unit than they are on the team nursing unit; more nursing time is logged with patients with a terminal prognosis if nurses are exposed to a workshop on the nursing care of the dying; baccalaureate-prepared nurses have a more democratic leadership style than diploma-prepared nurses. However, the work does not stop with the answers to the research questions; the investigator must also apply the answers to the research problem and say what they mean in terms of the problem, and that requires interpretation of the findings. First, though, we will talk about data analysis, how to get the findings, mostly in terms of the first step in data analysis, which is the development of categories.

DEVELOPING CATEGORIES OF RESPONSE

There are some rules about how categories are developed, and although there is underlying agreement about what the rules are, different authors talk about them in different ways (Fox, 1969; Kerlinger, 1973; Selltiz et al., 1966). We will follow Kerlinger (1973), who tells us that the investigator categorizes sets of objects by partitioning the responses, that is, by breaking down the responses into their constituent parts, according to some rule. The rule tells how to assign the objects to the partitions. What would the "partitions" be for a set of responses to a question about the gender of the subjects? Right! The responses would be partitioned into a category called "Male" and a category called "Female." What are the constituent parts of Grade Status? How about our old friends: A, B, C, D, F? The responses are partitioned, or grouped, according to the attributes of the variable.

The research question or the hypothesis tested in the study provides a basis for selecting the *principles of classification* for the category sets (Selltiz et al., 1966). In the classification process, the investigator assigns each response to one or more of a set of categories (Fox, 1969).

The categories themselves are structured according to some rules. Kerlinger (1973) identifies five rules for the development of categories.

1. *Categories must be set up according to the research problem and purpose.* Kerlinger says that this is the most important requirement, since if the categories are not set up in this

way, there is no answer obtained for the research questions; that is, the findings will not be relevant to the question asked. Fox (1969) presents this concept as a matter of *homogeneity*, which demands that all the categories bear a logical relationship to the variable of interest, and to one another, and of *usefulness*, which demands that each category serve a purpose and provide meaningful dimensions of the variable under study. He offers an example of homogeneity. If the investigator is partitioning responses (categorizing) on the basis of eye color of subjects and has a category set consisting of the categories of Blue-Eyed, Brown-Eyed, Black-Eyed, and Green-Eyed, he has a homogeneous set. If Nearsighted is added as a category partition, the homogeneity of the set is destroyed.

A study by Priscilla Mullins, in which she looks at the relationship between patient satisfaction and the type of delivery of nursing care, provides an example of category development. *Type of Delivery of Nursing Care* is partitioned into two categories: Team Nursing and Primary Nursing. The population consists of the patients on two large units (Team Nursing Unit and Primary Care Nursing Unit) at the time the data are collected. The sample consists of a random selection of 50 patients from each of the units, who will volunteer to be in the study. The study is straightforward and provides information from the patients as to how many of them are satisfied with the nursing care. The responses to the question "Are you satisfied with the nursing care?" are categorized as Satisfied and Not Satisfied. "Yes" responses are put in the Satisfied category and "no" responses are put in the Not Satisfied category. She can juxtapose, that is, put together, the variables as follows.

	SATISFIED	NOT SATISFIED
Primary Unit	40	10
Team Unit	20	30

She puts the numbers into the cells. The numbers in the cells are how many subjects said "yes" and how many subjects said "no" on each unit. *Cells* are the spaces where the two variables come together. Satisfied, Primary Unit is a cell with 40 responses; Not Satisfied, Primary Unit is a cell with 10 responses; Satisfied, Team Unit is a cell with 20 responses; Not Satisfied, Team Unit is a cell with 30 responses. She has developed a 2 × 2 frequency distribution, and she can carry out statistical manipulations on her cell frequencies such that she can answer the question of whether there is a relationship between patient satisfaction and type of delivery of nursing care.

If she had interval level data, perhaps from a satisfaction scale, that would give her some scores for each subject, she would have a different analytic paradigm, a different model, that would look like this:

PRIMARY NURSING	TEAM NURSING
60	30
54	39
28	29
"	"
"	"
"	"

The numbers are scores on the scale, and she would have 50 of them in each column. She could get an average score and do a statistical test to find out if the average satisfaction score for the Primary Unit is greater than the average satisfaction score for the Team Unit. She would be answering the same research question as she did in the previous example: Is the type of delivery of nursing care related to patient satisfaction?

Priscilla Mullins is a head nurse and is interested in relationships between patient satisfaction and system of delivery of nursing care. Because she knows that other variables might also have an impact on patient satisfaction, she collects data on the level of education and the marital status of the nurses and the medical diagnoses of the patients. It is clearly necessary that she build nursing education and medical diagnoses into her model, since these might interact with type of delivery of care to influence patient satisfaction scores. She would have more than one independent variable and would need to build a different model, which would still be based on her research question. However, adding marital status of nurses to her model would not be a good idea, since this probably does not fit into her research purpose. How much nurses know and how sick patients are, are plausible factors to consider in patient satisfaction with care. Whether nurses are married does not appear relevant to this study.

2. *Categories are exhaustive.* This means that all the responses of the subjects must be used up (Kerlinger, 1973, p. 138); that is, there has to be some place to put every response. In the Mullins' study, all the nurses must be either team nurses or primary nurses. It is not unheard of for a team unit to revert to functional nursing at 11 PM; if this happens, Mullins needs another category called Team plus Functional, or Mixed, and will probably have to ask her satisfaction questions according to shifts. If the unit is only a team unit from 8 to 8, she would not really be answering her research question if she left out the influence of the night nurses. In order for the category set for her independent variable to be exhaustive (include all the types of delivery of care), she would have to find some pure units or add a category called Mixed Unit.

Fox (1969) calls this *inclusiveness* and says that the set of categories must allow for all possible variations and permit every response to be classified. He would allow the use of a category called Miscellaneous (or Other) but points out that if the miscellaneous category catches more than 10 per cent of the responses, something is wrong with the set; the categories probably do not reflect the research question.

3. *Categories are mutually exclusive and independent. Mutually exclusive* means that each subject, or rather the *measure* assigned to each subject, must be clearly assignable to one cell and only one cell. The investigator who has clear operational definitions of the variables can do this. If the variable "level of education" is partitioned as "degree nurse/non-degree nurse," it must be quite clear what is meant by "degree nurse." Does that mean everyone but diploma-prepared nurses? How would a diploma nurse with a baccalaureate degree in business administration be assigned? Or a nurse with an associate arts degree? Priscilla Mullins must clarify: a degree nurse is a registered nurse with a baccalaureate degree in nursing. Every subject in the sample with these credentials of licensure and education is a degree nurse for the study; every other subject is assigned to the non-degree category.

Fox (1969) also calls this *mutual exclusiveness* and says that each category must represent one unique dimension of the variable under study.

Independent says that assignment to one cell does not affect assignment to another cell in the model; this is difficult to control, but random assignment to groups is expected to do it. If an academic investigator wanted to compare computer instruction with lecture in terms of motivating registered nurses to do research (what is the impact of mode of instruction on motivation to do research?), he should not allow subjects to select themselves into the two teaching groups. Self-selection may allow all the subjects with the highest motivation to choose the computer group, so that assignment to the computer teacher also means "assignment to" a high level of motivation to do research. A clear example of categories that are mutually exclusive, but *not* independent, is found in the sets Gender (Male/Female) and Pregnancy Status (Pregnant/Not Pregnant). A subject assigned to the category Male is automatically assigned to the category Not Pregnant; thus the two cells are not independent of each other.

4. *Each category must derive from only one classification principle.* This means that each variable must be treated at a separate level in the analytic paradigm because each variable is a separate dimension (Kerlinger, 1973). The investigator cannot put two variables in one category. This is simpler than it sounds, when the paradigm is examined. Let us look at the Mullins study of primary and team nursing.

She has two units that are pure units, where primary and team nursing occur on all three shifts, and patient satisfaction scores from each unit. She also has level of education of the nurses. What if she set up her analysis paradigm like this ?

	SATISFIED	NOT SATISFIED
Primary		
Team		
Degree		
No Degree		

Does she have a good model? Obviously not, and the reason is that the categories of her independent variables are not derived from one classification principle, but two. Where does she put a check mark for the satisfied patient on the primary unit whose nurse does not have a degree? She needs a better model in which each independent variable has a principle all its own and a category level all its own. It would probably look like this:

	SATISFIED		NOT SATISFIED	
	Primary	*Team*	*Primary*	*Team*
Degree				
No Degree				

Every variable is derived from one classification principle, and Priscilla Mullins has a place for all her responses.

5. *Any categorization scheme must have one level of discourse.* Kerlinger (1973) says that this is the hardest rule to define, and he defines it in terms of set theory. Fortunately, he also discusses it in terms of dependent measures. The rules for the development of categories defined earlier are about how to partition independent variables. The level of discourse rule is concerned with dependent measures; the universe of discourse is the set of dependent variable measures. If the investigator switches to a different kind of dependent variable, then the level of discourse is changed. If Priscilla Mullins is interested in patient satisfaction as a dependent variable and is happily looking for relationships between patient satisfaction and different nurse variables (years of experience, for instance, or type of delivery of care, or level of education), she cannot suddenly begin to include nursing performance in her dependent variable measure. If the dependent measure is patient satisfaction, that is what she must address. If it suddenly occurs to her that the independent variables (years of experience and level of education) might also have some effect on nursing performance, which is another dependent variable, she has switched her level of discourse.

Now, there is nothing to prevent her from measuring more than one dependent variable, or from addressing an intervening variable, that is, a variable that may come between the independent variable and the dependent variable, and in some way mediate the effect of one on the other. She can look at the relationships between years of experience, level of education, and nursing performance and then look at the impact of nursing performance on patient satisfaction, but it must be clear what she is doing and her analytic paradigm must indicate the separate dimensions of the variables. She must not, without warning, in the discussion section of her report, throw in the impact of education on nursing performance if she hasn't brought nursing performance up before and built it into her design.

Some investigators, when they do not find the expected relationships between the independent variables and the dependent variables, talk a lot about a relationship they just happened to find between the independent variable and another dependent variable. Priscilla Mullins would never do that because she knows the rules. This is not to say that serendipitous findings, which are unexpected and happy things that show up when the investigator is looking for something else, should not be presented; they most certainly should, but they should not contaminate and confuse the categorization scheme. To go back to an earlier example about eye color, the investigator cannot just throw nearsightedness into the discussion, although it could be built in as another measure of interest, if the formulation of the problem would allow it.

STATISTICAL MANIPULATION

Do not stop reading because you never understood arithmetic. This is not about arithmetic; it is about some more rules you need to understand in order to get a little information from the tables most investigators provide for you in their research reports. You already know that 3 is more than 2, and that the space between 2 and 3 is the same as the space between 1 and 2, and that .30 is less than .90. You have already learned a lot about the steps in the research process. You know more than you think you do about statistical concepts, and you are going to learn just a little more. As a practitioner in a science-based profession, you must understand the meaning of some terms, since scientists try to quantify their results. Some of the terms may appear ominous to you, but do not panic; there will be no arithmetic in this explanation. The discussion remains elementary; when you are ready to move beyond that, the explanations of the concepts will be full of formulae, and you will enjoy that too.

The first thing to consider in statistical manipulation of the data is, why do it anyhow? Why not talk about it all in words rather than in numbers? Since the interpretation of the findings is in words at the last, why ever leave the words for the numbers? Think back to generalization: remember, the investigator usually wants to say something about a population on the basis of the behavior of a sample. In order to make statements about a population, the investigator probably must summarize the findings from many individual measures. If the investigator wants to determine whether baccalaureate nurses show a different pattern of adaptation to caring for patients in the home setting than do non-baccaluareate nurses, many subjects from each population will be selected to measure. What will he do with 1,000 "adaptation to home nursing" scores from each group? You know the answer to that, even if you do not like arithmetic. He will get an *average* score for each group; that is, he will summarize the individual measures, typify the twc collections of 1,000 measures, each with a single number, one for each collection. He can do more. He can see if the difference in the averages is likely to be a chance difference; that is, he can *estimate the probability* that the difference between the averages of the scores will occur again in another set of individual measures from the same population. As an investigator, he wants to say that the difference is the result of real differences in the subjects on the variable of adaptation. Statistical manipulation gives him ways to do this, or, of course, of finding out that it *is* all due to chance. Investigators* using statistics may be interested simply in describing the characteristics of a group and will use *descriptive* statistics to do so. Or they may be interested in the characteristics of a larger group, a population, and use the findings from a smaller group, a sample, to make inferences about the characteristics of the larger group. Now that is something you already knew: the added information is that certain techniques, called sampling or *inferential* statistics, are used in generalizing from the sample to the population. These are frequently the same statistics, the same formulae, as the statistics used in descriptive work, but the function of the statistics is not the same.

Purposes of Statistical Manipulation

The function of descriptive statistics is the organization and description of large collections of numbers, and there are several uses to be considered.

Organizing Data. A frequency distribution is developed to organize the data. In a collection of 1,000 scores ranging from 1 to 100, how many subjects scored 1, how many scored 2, how many scored 3... how many scored 100? That is, what is the frequency of occurrence for each score? This is a *unit* frequency distribution. With 1,000 scores to deal with, the investigator

---

*This chapter depends on notes freely adapted through 15 years of teaching, which were originally freely adapted from Chapter 34 in the 1964 edition of *Foundations of Behavioral Research*, by Fred N. Kerlinger. Although the concepts are all addressed by Kerlinger, he should not be held responsible for the simplification in the presentation, and therefore, he is not referenced in the usual manner in this portion of the text.

would be more likely to establish a *group* frequency distribution and establish how many subjects scored between 1 and 10, how many scored between 11 and 20, how many scored between 21 and 30 ... how many scored between 91 and 100. Now do not go away thinking that all group distributions have an interval of 10; the interval size can be whatever is appropriate.

Picturing Data. The investigator can organize the data into graphs, which are visual frequency distributions. You know what a bar graph is; remember your lectures on nutrition, with all the sources of vitamins and minerals compared with bar graphs of different colors? The lengths of the bars in the graph represent the amount of the variable present. There are other kinds of visual frequency distributions; frequency polygons, which are single lines drawn from point to point, and histograms, which are classy bar graphs used for ratio level data.

Describing Data Numerically

Measures of Central Tendency. Sometimes the investigator wants to describe a data set with one number, to typify the set of scores with the score most like the others in that set. He will use the average score, the measure of central tendency. There are several measures of central tendency, *averages*, and we will consider three of them: the arithmetic mean, the median, and the mode. When the investigator wants to typify an entire collection of numbers with a single number, that is, to use one score as the typical score, he will use the average score for the group. If he has interval or ratio level data, he may choose the arithmetic mean, which is the sum of all the scores divided by the number of the scores. If he has ordinal level data, ranked data, he may choose the median, the point on the scale of scores below which one-half the scores fall. If he has only nominal data, categorical data, he must choose the mode, which is the most frequently occurring score. Actually, he has little choice, since he cannot use the arithmetic mean unless he has certain levels of data. He can always go down and use a median or a mode for interval data, but he cannot step up and use an arithmetic mean for nominal or ordinal level data.

Sometimes, though, even if he has interval level data, he may be better off using the median, rather than the arithmetic mean, if there are scores that are very high or very low compared with the rest of the scores. Keep in mind that he is trying to find one score that will *typify* the entire collection of scores. A very high score or a very low score pulls the arithmetic mean in the direction of that score, since the magnitude of all the scores is represented in this measure. The median looks at how the scores are ranked, rather than at the absolute magnitude of the individual scores, and may better represent what most of the scores are.

For example, seven persons run the 100-yard dash. The length of time in seconds it took each person was 11.0, 11.0,

11.0, 11.2, 11.6, 12.1, 17.1. The arithmetic mean can be obtained for time data; for this set of scores, it is 12.14. The median is 11.2. Which number best typifies this set of scores? Right, the median. Although the level of the data allows the use of the more powerful statistic, the less powerful statistic would be used. In order to know which measure of central tendency to use, given a choice, the investigator asks the question of how well the score describes the rest of the scores.

Measures of Variability. Along with knowing the typical score, the investigator wants to know how the scores are dispersed, the range of the scores. In its simplest form, this is the line from the lowest score to the highest score, and this is the form used when the measure of central tendency is the mode. When the average is the median, it should be accompanied by a more sophisticated statement of variability, called the semi-interquartile range. When the arithmetic mean is calculated, the calculation of a precise and elegant statement of dispersion, called the standard deviation, is also done. You will be happy to know that we are not going to figure any of these. But you must remember that which measure of central tendency is calculated depends on the level of the data first and on the characteristics of the scores second, and that each measure of central tendency (average) has its own measure of the dispersion of the scores around the mean, the variability of the scores.

Shape Characteristics. Shape characteristics are how the data would look if they were graphed. It is frequently useful to the statistician to know the *shape of the distribution* in terms of its lateral symmetry—its deviations from center—and the flatness or peakedness of the curve. The names for these two shape characteristics are *skewness* and *kurtosis*, just in case you run across them. In order to understand them, we would need to get into some heavy numbers and heavy breathing, and indeed, some advanced methods texts do not give you much more information than this. If you want to worry about the shape of the curve, you will want to purchase a statistics text and an advanced methods text. For our purposes, remember that sometimes the shape of the distribution of the data provides useful information.

Interpreting Individual Values Among Data. Sometimes the investigator wants to know how an individual score stands in relation to the whole score set, and there are many techniques to help with this. *Percentiles* and *standard scores* are two commonly used techniques. A percentile is the score below which a given percentages of the scores fall. Many test results, for instance, the College Board Examination (CBE), are represented in percentiles. If you scored on the CBE in the 82d percentile, this means that your score was the same or better than the scores of 82 per cent of the test takers. Standard scores have been rescaled so that the mean is 0 and the standard deviation is 1. This is done so that scores from different distributions may be compared.

Making Correlations. Sometimes the investigator wants to describe the relationships between two or more sets of scores. Both the magnitude and the direction of the relationships can be provided by a whole set of statistical techniques known as correlation techniques.

Choice of Statistical Techniques

All the techniques described are also used in inferential statistics, as well as many that are not mentioned here. The rules for when you can use what are different: if you want to use inferential statistics, that is, if you want to generalize the sample findings to a population, certain requirements must be met as to how data are collected and how subjects are selected into the sample.

For the investigator, the choice of a statistical technique depends on several things. The way the question is asked, in terms of a relationship or a difference, and the type of scale formed by the data, i.e., the level of the data, influence the choice. Because some statistics are appropriate for small samples and some are not, the size of the sample must be considered. Design questions (for instance, whether the measures are related—that is, same subject, time one and time two—or independent—that is, different groups of subjects) must also be considered. If statistics comparing averages are used, which is not unlikely, the investigator should provide the reader with at least three pieces of information about the data: the number of cases, that is, the size of the sample; the measure of central tendency, that is, the average; and the variability of the scores, that is, some numerical statement about the range. This information, plus the data collection technique, will allow the reader to consider whether the statistics are appropriate. If you are still unwilling to address the numbers, be calm; you can usually depend on the editors of the research journals to screen the statistics.

Types of Statistical Presentations

There are several main types of statistical presentations, and we will look at a few of them here.

Frequency Distribution. This may be primary or secondary. In the primary frequency distribution, the presentation is simply the number of cases falling into each category. If you toss a penny 20 times and keep track of the number of times it falls heads up and the number of times it falls tails up, you have generated a primary frequency distribution. In a secondary frequency distribution, you juxtapose the categories of variables so that relationships can be studied. Priscilla Mullins did that when she was studying the influence of systems of care on patient satisfaction.

Measures of Central Tendency. These are *averages*, typical scores, and may be used in other statistical techniques to compare groups of measures (is the difference between the mean of Group

1 and the mean of Group 2 statistically significant?); to represent all the measures in the group with one number; and to interpret individual scores (how close is a given score to the mean?).

Variability of a Set of Measures. The variability of the scores is concerned with how close or how far they are from the mean score; if an investigator reports a mean, he should also report the appropriate variability. The mean score for a group of five students, all of whom score 3 on a 5-point test, is 3. The mean score for a group of 5 students, who score respectively, 1, 2, 3, 4, 5 on a 5-point test is also 3. However, the members of the two groups probably have different knowledge levels; in order to counsel for the next test, the teacher needs to know the variability.

Measures of Relations. There are many measures of relations, and they all do the same thing: they tell if a relationship exists between variables. Some of them, called *coefficients of correlation*, also tell the *degree* of the association.

Analyses of Differences. When the investigator is interested in whether two groups are different, rather than whether they are associated, there are statistical techniques which examine the differences between groups. Remember that the hypothesis can be a prediction of a relationship or of a difference. How the hypothesis is stated is one of the elements in the design that has an impact on the kind of statistical technique chosen.

Many more kinds of statistical presentations of data are possible: we have covered the ones you are most likely to see in your reading. As a final word, a course in statistics is more fun than you might think and certainly will be useful to you in your reading. If your curriculum does not require it, ask for it as an elective and shake up your adviser.

INTERPRETATION OF THE FINDINGS

Analysis by itself does not provide answers to research questions; it provides *findings*, the results of the categorization and statistical manipulation of the data. The investigator must also *interpret*, explain the findings, and find meaning in them.

Two kinds of interpretation may be attempted. A narrow search for the meaning of the findings within the bounds of the study may be made; Group 1 is different from Group 2 in this population in this setting, and decisions on the basis of the findings are made within the population and the setting. There is no intent to say that the differences are relevant to any other population and setting. The investigator may, however, be interested in seeking a broader meaning in the findings and say that the difference between Group 1 and Group 2 is relevant to other populations and settings. If this is the case, he will compare his results with other research results from the literature and/or with the expectations of the theory he is testing with his hypotheses.

He will say things like, "The difference in these groups supports the results reported by Smith and Jones in their seminal studies; however, the results of this study are in disagreement with Robinson's findings. The original Robinson study is, of course, faulted for inappropriate sampling, but his results have been replicated in several instances (see notes on the Robinson graduate student studies)." The investigator must lodge himself and his findings in the literature about the variables he has studied and find the meaning of his results in that literature.

A critical reader of research will carry out his own interpretive activities as he decides whether the investigator can attribute all that much meaning to the findings. The reader who understands the steps in the research process will evaluate the technical soundness of the design and ask first if the results are based in sound design and can therefore be trusted. Given that the results are trustworthy, is it logical and plausible to believe that they mean what the investigator says they mean? If the answer to all the above is "yes," then nursing practice may be adjusted on the basis of the findings.

A final word about findings. It is easy enough to assign meaning to positive findings (the researcher found what he expected to find, on the basis of the empirical literature and the theories of interest, and explains the findings out of the theory and the literature), but how are negative or inconclusive findings to be interpreted? What do they mean?

Such results can be useful in science, although it is not easy to get them published. Negative results can be caused by four factors—incorrect theory or hypotheses, inappropriate or incorrect methods, inadequate or poor measurement and faulty analysis—or any combination of these. If none of the last three factors is faulty, if the methodology is appropriate and correct, the measurement is adequate and good, and the analysis impeccable, then what is left may be an incorrect theory or hypotheses not based in the theory. It is surely a contribution to science to point out that a theory isn't working as well as it is supposed to when it is tested in real life, or that hypotheses that are supposed to be derived from the theory do not seem to be predicting anything they should. The point to be made in this book is that negative and inconclusive results do not of themselves indicate wrongness in the investigative activity, or "poor" research: they can be as useful to the science and to the practice as positive findings, although they are more difficult to interpret. Another point for this book, and for the person who is learning from it what goes into a critical review, is that interpretation does not stop with the investigator: the reader is as critical of the interpretation as of the rest of the study, giving credit where it is due but not assuming that the meaning assigned to the findings by the author is the only meaning to be found, the best meaning to be found, or even there at all. The critical reader keeps asking if the investigator can, in logic, get to the meaning from the findings. The two questions are always there: Are the results based on sound methodology? and Is the interpretation of the results logical and plausible?

SUMMARY

The steps *data analysis* and *data interpretation* constitute the interpretive phase of the research activity. Data analysis is the *categorization* of the data, using rules of category development, followed by *statistical manipulation*.

Categories must *reflect the research problem*, and be *exhaustive*, *mutually exclusive*, and *independent*; they also must be derived from *one classification principle*. A category scheme must have only *one level of discourse*.

The statistical manipulation is done to *organize data* into frequency distributions, *picture data* in graphs or polygons, *describe data numerically*, for instance, obtain means and standard deviations, and *interpret individual values* or establish *correlations* or differences among the variables.

Interpretation of the data establishes the *meaning* of the findings, either broadly in terms of the research problem or narrowly within the bounds of the study.

References

Fox, D.J. The Research Process in Education. New York: Holt, Rinehart & Winston, 1969.
Kerlinger, F.N. Foundations of Behavioral Research. New York: Holt, Rinehart & Winston, 1964.
Kerlinger, F.N. Foundations of Behavioral Research. 2d ed. New York: Holt, Rinehart & Winston, 1973.
Selltiz, C., M. Jahoda, M. Deutsch, and S.W. Cook. Research Methods in Social Relations. New York: Holt, Rinehart & Winston, 1966.

Study Activities

1. Differentiate *data analysis* and *data interpretation*.

2. List the rules for categorization, and provide an example for each rule.

3. List the functions of descriptive statistics as these are developed in the text, and provide an example for each function.

4. Differentiate *descriptive statistics* and *inferential statistics*.
5. List several types of statistical presentations, and provide an example of each type.
6. Describe the kinds of interpretation that may be attempted by the investigator.
7. Describe how the investigator seeks a broad meaning of the findings.

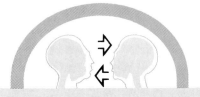

11

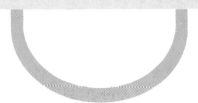

When you complete Chapter 11, you will be able to...

1. Describe the three basic principles identified in the Belmont Report.

2. Describe the three requirements in the conduct of research that evolve from the principles.

3. Describe the elements of informed consent.

ETHICAL CONSIDERATIONS

Heretofore we have been concerned with factors of technical soundness in the research plan and the data-collection and analysis techniques and with the logic of the data interpretation. In this chapter, the assumptions of appropriate methodology and appropriate interpretation will be made, and attention will be focused on some ethical considerations in research.

Now, this is more complex than you might think. You know already, from comments in earlier chapters, that subjects in research studies have *human rights* that must be considered by the investigators. Investigators have rights too; perhaps we can call them scientific rights. Investigators also have scientific obligations, as well as responsibilities to protect their subjects, and this set of rights, obligations, and responsibilities in the two groups of people are intertwined and interrelated.

The rights of investigators grow out of the societal mandate to develop the science and the practice. Because society requires scientists to advance their science, some rights to the activities inherent in advancement necessarily accrue. The expansion of scientific knowledge *requires* the activities of research, and as Gray (1975) points out, the ethical problems generated by experimentation with human subjects cannot be evaded by refusing to select subjects from human populations, since the failure to pursue knowledge of possible benefit to society may itself be unethical when such pursuit is desirable. He also points out, more pragmatically, that in many clinical settings, the distinction between experimentation and treatment is problematic.

The American Nurses' Association *Human Rights Guidelines*

for Nurses in Clinical and Other Research (1985) identifies human rights in two sets of people, the researchers and the subjects. The document speaks to the rights of qualified nurses to do research and to access resources to implement scientific investigations; also, the document clarifies the rights of persons who are recipients of health care or participants in research that impinges on the patient care provided by nurses. When nursing activities are performed by nurses as part of a clinical research design, the protection of human rights extends to the nurses who do as well as to the subjects who are done to. The nurses who are part of the manipulation of the independent variable or who serve as data collectors, as well as the patients who are subjects, are entitled to the options spelled out by regulations for the development of ethical design.

There is a moral obligation to seek new knowledge, but it is never separate from a moral obligation always to consider the rights of the subjects who are expected to provide the new knowledge. The investigator is in a relationship of trust with his subjects. When the investigator is a nurse and the subjects are patients, the responsibility is more than doubled. It is not only that nurses purport to be patients' advocates, and therefore their protectors from the dangers of experiment; it is that the researcher also has a responsibility to the research design, which must be considered. The two responsibilities are frequently in conflict in clinical and behavioral science research. A researcher is committed to furthering knowledge rather than to meeting individual patient needs. Thus, although the *researcher/subject* role and the *nurse/patient* role are both based in trust, when patient needs are in conflict with the requirements of the research design, the nurse investigator is in a professional dilemma.

Because this book is concerned with the education of critical consumers of research, rather than with the education of principal investigators, this chapter addresses the regulations designed for the protection of the rights of research subjects, rather than the rights and conflicting responsibilities of investigators. The critical reader looks for some statement from the investigator indicating how the rights of subjects were protected and considers ethical soundness as well as technical soundness in designs.

The current consideration for the rights of subjects began after knowledge of the dreadful experimentation that was made public in the Nuremberg trials, and that resulted in the development of the Nuremberg Code, a set of 10 principles related to human experimentation. The Code is the first effort to establish principles and guidelines for human experimentation, Many later codes use the principles, particularly the material contained in the first clause, which has to do with the voluntary consent of subjects. The Code has a major fault, however, in that it depends on *self-regulation* by the experimenter (Fromer, 1981). Unfortunately, a large body of evidence suggests that experimenters cannot always be depended on to attend to the protection of their subjects (Pappworth, 1967; Gray, 1975; Brandt, 1978; Rothman, 1982). Various organizational and governmental documents reflect the need for further development of protective and regulatory principles.

Reports in the national, rather than the scientific, press have called attention to clinical and behavioral studies of questionable ethical caliber. In the Tuskegee syphilis study, researchers inhibited the treatment of venereal disease in a population of black males in order to continue a study of the natural progress of the disease. This study, which was begun in 1932, was not discontinued until 1972. It was carried out under the auspices of the venereal disease division of the United States Public Health Service and reported frequently in the medical literature. It was clear from the reports that medical attention for the disease was denied the subjects, although the efficacy of penicillin was established and the Nuremberg Code was in place. In the Willowbrook study, an equally questionable effort, a research team, over a period of years, systematically inoculated groups of new residents admitted to an institution for the mentally retarded with hepatitis viruses. This work was also reported in the scientific literature. The investigators involved have defended both of the projects ably and insist that the research protocols were ethical (Rothman, 1982).

These were clinical studies; there were also studies reported from the social sciences that led to fervent discussion of the ethical parameters of investigator manipulation of independent variables. In this atmosphere of concern for the human rights of subjects by the public as well as by some scientists, the 1974 Congress passed a National Research Act (Public Law 93-348), which established the National Commission for the Protection of Human Subjects of Biomedical and Behavioral Research. The Commission was charged with the development of ethical guidelines for the conduct of research involving human subjects and with making recommendations to the Secretary of Health, Education and Welfare, with respect to research conducted, supported, or regulated by the Department of Health, Education and Welfare (DHEW), and to Congress, with respect to research not subject to DHEW regulation. The history of the activities of the Commission and of the recommendations submitted and the regulations promulgated is extremely interesting and useful to an investigator coming to terms with the rights of subjects. Two sources of information are the transcript of several public hearings held by the Commission (PB-270 258, US Department of Commerce, 1977) and The New Federal Regulations: What They Do or Do Not Regulate (PRIM & R, 1981).

THE BELMONT REPORT

The critical reader can be satisfied with knowing the principles and guidelines for the protection of human subjects recommended by the Commission, as presented in the Belmont Report (1978), since these constitute the basis of the various protective procedures now used.

The Belmont Report distinguishes between research and practice, develops discussion around three basic ethical principles, and addresses some considerations in application of the principles. The distinction made between research and practice is useful to nurses and other clinical groups, since in clinical settings the distinction is not always clear. For instance, the final step of the nursing process is Evaluation, and there is frequently a question as to when the evaluation of nursing interventions is a research rather than a practice activity, and thereby subject to review as a research protocol. The Commissioners differentiate research from practice in terms of the reason for the activity: practice refers to interventions that are designed solely to enhance the well-being of an individual patient or client and that have a reasonable expectation of success. The purpose is to help the client. Research designates activities designed to develop or contribute to generalizable knowledge. Innovative treatment is not, of itself, research. They say that research and practice may be carried on together, in evaluating the safety or efficacy of a therapy, but if there is any question as to whether there is an element of research present in the activity, that activity should undergo review for the protection of subjects.

Basic Principles of Ethical Research

The Belmont Report identifies three basic principles as relevant to the ethics of research involving human subjects: respect for persons, beneficence, and justice.

Respect for Persons. The principle of respect for persons involves two convictions: individuals are autonomous and the autonomy should be respected; and persons with diminished autonomy require protection. Human subjects should always enter into a study voluntarily and with information adequate for the decision to participate or not to participate in the research. However, vulnerable populations who may not really have decision-making powers (for instance, prisoners, students, patients, the very young, and the very old) require special protection, to inhibit coercion or undue influence on the part of investigators or their friends in administration.

Beneficence. The principle of beneficence involves an effort to secure the well-being of persons. It is understood as an obligation in the Belmont Report, and the investigator is expected not to do harm and to maximize possible benefits and minimize possible harms to subjects.

Justice. The third principle is justice. Justice is concerned with the systematic selection of various groups as human subjects. Selection that is associated with easy availability, or ease of manipulation owing to institutional or minority status, or economic class, or to other variables not related to the research is addressed in the application of this principle.

Requirements of Ethical Research

The Commissioners considered that three requirements in the conduct of research evolve from the three principles identified. The requirements are *informed consent, risk/benefit assessment,* and the *fair selection of subjects.*

Informed Consent. Respect for persons requires that all individuals have the opportunity to choose what shall or shall not happen to them; this principle is satisfied when requirements for informed consent are met. Informed consent is considered to contain three elements: *information, comprehension,* and *voluntariness.*

Information identifies specific items of the research process for disclosure by the investigator to the potential subjects. Generally, these items include the research procedure, the purpose of the research, possible risks and anticipated benefits, and alternative procedures if therapy is involved. Subjects should be informed that they need not volunteer and may withdraw at any time, and they should be offered an opportunity to ask questions.

It is always a difficult decision for the investigator as to what is appropriate to tell potential subjects, but it is especially difficult when providing the information impairs the integrity of the design. Incomplete disclosure *may* be justified if it is truly necessary to accomplish the research goal, there are no undisclosed risks to the subjects, and there are plans for debriefing when the study is completed. However, some people believe that incomplete disclosure is never justified.

Comprehension is concerned with the manner in which information is conveyed and the subjects' ability to understand the information. The investigator must be sure that the subjects comprehend the material, and she must guard against a merely legalistic presentation of a list of items. For those special instances when subject selection is from a noncomprehending population (e.g., subjects who are mentally disabled, very young, very old, or comatose), a proxy consent may be provided by a responsible third party. However, such subjects should be provided with information and be encouraged to exercise decision-making powers to the best of their abilities to comprehend and to decide, and the investigator must be able to justify their use as subjects in terms of the requirements of the study, rather than because of their availability.

Voluntariness indicates that consent is valid only if it is a free choice. Procedures for obtaining consent must be free of coercion and undue influence. Potential subjects may not be threatened into consent, nor can they be offered excessive rewards for consent.

Risk-Benefit Assessment. This assessment justifies the research in relation to the principle of beneficence. Risk refers to a possibility that harm may occur because of participation in the research and is used to describe the severity of the possible harm. Benefit is concerned with the positive values provided by the research. Risks and benefits may affect individual subjects, their families, special groups of subjects, or the larger society.

The assessment is qualitative as a rule, although it is common to refer to a "favorable risk-benefit ratio" as though quantitative analysis is always done. It is not, but some systematic analysis is always possible. This will include assessment of the validity and significance of the research and the nature, probability, and magnitude of the risks.

Fair Selection. The principle of justice requires that there are fair procedures and outcomes in the selection of subjects. It is not appropriate to offer selection into beneficial research to "desirable" persons and selection into risky studies to "undesirable" persons. It is not correct that certain classes of persons bear the burden of participation in research because they are in a powerless condition. Subjects who are in a dependent status must be protected against the danger of being involved in research simply for the convenience of the investigator or because they can be manipulated owing to their dependency.

RIGHTS OF HUMAN SUBJECTS

The federal government continues to take an interest in the rights of human subjects, and since it is the major funding agency for clinical and behavioral studies, the regulations promulgated for the protection of human subjects in federally funded research are, as a rule, adopted by institutions for all research carried out under institutional auspices.

Responsibility for the protection of subjects lies permanently and primarily with the investigator: the obligation is both moral and legal. The submission of the research protocol for review by a committee of peers is a protection for the investigator and for the sponsoring agency, as well as for the subjects.

Examination of research proposals using human subjects is carried out through the deliberations of Institutional Review Boards (IRBs) of one kind or another. The existence of such a board to review human subject research proposals is frequently a requirement for federal funding of any sort for the institution. Although board membership and board activities are defined in various ways in the different settings, hospital boards are likely to be composed of physicians. University boards usually are more diverse in membership, with some effort made to include representatives from all the relevant sciences as well as an outside membership representing the public and the law.

The purpose of the IRBs is to protect subjects from their investigators and from the risks imposed by the research design. They represent the institution that must authorize implementation of the research.

Many research studies are exempted from review by the institution's IRB: for example, studies dealing with normal educational practices; surveys or interviews or observations of public behavior that do not identify subjects or place them at risk, or that do not involve sensitive behavior; the use of available data, such as records, reports, or diagnostic specimens. Also, expedited review, that is, examination of the research protocol by one or two members of the IRB, may be carried out for certain studies dealing with routine noninvasive procedures, healthy autonomous subjects, or the use of discarded body tissues. However, even if studies are exempt or receive expedited review, the responsibility of the *investigator* to protect subjects does not change.

Ethical Issues That Should Be Addressed in Research Reports

Part of the critical review is the evaluation of the ethical parameters of a particular design, and the investigator should provide the information necessary for evaluation. Sometimes this is done simply by noting that the study has been through an IRB review; however, a few paragraphs mentioning the matters of most importance to the subjects in the specified study are of more use to the reader.

The critical reader of reports of studies in which samples were selected from human populations should have information from the investigator on three topics related to the protection of the subjects: invasion of privacy, the elements of informed consent, and some assessment of the risks of the study. The latter should also contain information concerning the benefits of the study to the individual subjects and to the science.

Invasion of Privacy. In a manner of speaking, any study invades the privacy of the subjects, since the invasion must occur simply for the investigator to ask the potential subject for permission to explain the study. Realistically, however, invasion of privacy becomes an issue when the research addresses sensitive variables. However, the subject should have the option of *not* hearing an explanation of the study, and it should be made clear in the study report that the option was offered.

Informed Consent. The need for the informed consent of the subject to experience the manipulation of the independent variables and the measurement of the dependent variables identified in the study is a major protection for human subjects. Brink and

Wood (1983) identify three major elements in informed consent: the type of information that should be provided by the investigator to the subjects; the degree of subject understanding of the parameters of the study and of investigator expectations for subject behaviors, which subjects must manifest; and subject autonomy in the setting in which consent is requested.

Type of Information Given to Subjects. Brink and Wood (1983) suggest a comprehensive list of items of subject information. It includes a statement in full detailing what will happen to subjects. The statement should include the nature, duration, and purpose of the study; the methods and procedures of data collection; some indication of how the data will be used; all the potential and actual inconveniences and risks to the subjects as a function of participation in the research; the benefits to be gained from participation; the subject's right not to participate and right to withdraw at any time; information concerning compensation for participation; and information concerning the treatment of injuries owing to participation.

Subjects' Understanding. There is more to informed consent than simply listing the information subjects should have before agreeing to participate in a study. The requirement is that the information must be presented in such a way that the subjects understand it; that is, it must be presented in the language of the subject, not the language of the science. There is evidence that this concept is not considered by many investigators, particularly in clinical settings, where the difficulty of describing the manipulation of the independent variable in lay terms is great (Gray, 1975). However difficult the task, it must be attempted and accomplished, and its accomplishment should be a part of the research report.

Subjects' Autonomy. It is the responsibility of the investigator to be sure that the subjects who are asked to participate in the study really do have the right to refuse to do so. Explicit coercion has become uncommon; there are few instances today of benefits being withheld *because* of refusal to participate in research. Implicit coercion is more common. Students participate in studies because teachers ask them to do so; patients participate in studies at the request of their physicians; institutionalized populations are not likely to say "no" when administrators in control of their lives are saying "yes." This kind of status coercion is hard to identify, since it is frequently not even identified by the subjects, but it must always be considered by the investigators. Subjects who do not themselves have the power to decide should not be asked to participate in studies.

The topic of the ethical implications in obtaining proxy consents for members of populations not of an age or a rational competence to understand the information provided is too complex for consideration in this book. The critical reader should require that the investigator provide explicit justification of such consents.

Risks to Subjects. Subjects have a right not to be harmed by the study, and although worthwhile designs that harbor risks to subjects will not be turned down by an IRB because of the risks, it rests with the investigator to explain why it is necessary to put subjects at risk. The information is given to the IRB and to the subjects involved. The investigator must justify risks in terms of benefits to accrue, and she must indicate how subjects are protected as much as possible. Protective measures may include previous studies in animal laboratories, plans for debriefing subjects after the study, and plans for providing control groups with the experimental treatment after the study is over. Risks may be other than physical in nature. Threats to self-worth, to values, and to privacy constitute risk, as do stressful study situations in which subjects are made anxious or embarrassed.

Two risks that are considered separately by IRBs are risks to confidentiality and to anonymity. Confidentiality is concerned with subjects' rights to have study information available only to the research team and not disseminated publicly. Anonymity is concerned with the rights of subjects not to be identified with their responses, or even to be identified as participants in the study. Both rights are protected by locking up data, by keeping master lists of subjects separated from the data responses, and by reticence on the part of the research team. The Friday night party is no place to share the funny answers the subjects provided to questions about sexuality.

Because data confidentiality has no legal standing, the protection of subjects who may be vulnerable to legal sanctions on the basis of their participation in the study may be particularly difficult. If such protection cannot be provided by the investigator, this information should be incorporated into the informed consent procedure.

Continuing Ethical Considerations in Research

There are no definitive solutions to the many ethical issues that arise in research with human subjects, although there is a continuing flow and revision of codes and regulations from government and professional organizations, addressing the generation of new knowledge without doing harm to human subjects. None of them answer the question of how high a probability of achieving how much benefit by a piece of research is necessary to justify exposing X number of human subjects to X level of risk (Gray, 1975, p. 3).

Pappworth (1967) identifies other faults in current ethical codes. They are not enforceable. They have no legal sanction.

There is much disagreement among the professionals affected by the codes concerning the need for and the content of the documents. Most codes are general and ambiguous in their wording. It is probably better to have them than not to have them, but the people most likely to follow codes probably are the people who do not really need them to behave in an ethical manner with subjects or clients. Pappworth (1967) suggests in his book of clinical studies that what is needed is a population of "real" volunteers, that is, persons who make a profession of being subjects in scientific experiments and are well paid for their efforts.

The studies designed by nurses are likely to contain all possible protection for their subjects. However, clinical nurses caring for patients who are selected into nursing and other studies have a responsibility to those patients that is part of nursing concern for their safety and well-being. Williamson (1981) says that nurses who are concerned for research threats to patient safety should make the concerns public. Nurses should remind patients of their rights to adequate information about proposed studies and support the patients' decisions, whatever these may be. She says that clinical nurses *involved* in research have certain rights: they must consent to participate, as do the patients/subjects. Once they decide to participate, they should really do so, keeping in touch with the principal investigator and reporting if the patients/subjects are not responding properly. This is also perceived as protecting the patients.

Williamson (1981) believes that the best protection the subject can have is good design, design that is scientifically sound and ethically sound. Ethical soundness is assured by IRB review of the proposal, by the informed consent of the subjects, obtained without coercion, by presentation of data in aggregate form, and protection of raw data from those who are not members of the research team.

SUMMARY

The critical reader asks the investigator for information as to how subjects have been protected from the requirements of the research design. This information should include how subjects were *selected* and asked to participate, what *information* they were given, what *choice* they had, how *confidentiality* and *anonymity* were maintained, what *risks* are identified, and how subjects were *protected against the risks. Benefits* expected from the findings may possibly be found in the paragraphs related to the significance of the study, but benefits should be made explicit also in the paragraphs devoted to the ethical dimensions of the study.

References

American Nurses' Association. Human Rights Guidelines for Nurses in Clinical and Other Research. D-46 5M. Kansas City, Mo.: American Nurses' Association, 1985.

Brandt, A.M. Racism and research: The case of the Tuskegee syphilis study. Hastings Center Report 6 (1978): 21-29.

Brink, P.J., and M.J. Wood. Basic Steps in Planning Nursing Research, from Question to Proposal. 2d ed. Monterey, Calif.: Wadsworth, 1983.

Fromer, M.J. Ethical Issues in Health Care. St. Louis: C.V. Mosby, 1981.

Gray, B.J. Human Subjects in Medical Experimentation. New York: John Wiley & Sons, 1975.

National Commission for the Protection of Human Subjects of Biomedical and Behavioral Research. The Belmont Report. DHEW Publication No. (OS) 78-0012. Washington, D.C.: Government Printing Office, 1978.

Pappworth, M.H. Human Guinea Pigs. Boston: Beacon Press, 1967.

Public Hearing on Institutional Review Boards. Transcript. Bethesda, Md.: National Commission for the Protection of Human Subjects in Biomedical and Behavioral Research (NTIS PB 270 258), 1977.

Rothman, D.J. Were Tuskegee and Willowbrook studies in nature? Hastings Center Report 2 (1982): 5-7.

The New Federal Regulations: What They Do and Do Not Regulate. Boston: Public Responsibility in Medicine and Research, 1981.

Williamson, Y.M. Ethics: Human subjects in research. In Y.M. Williamson, ed. Research Methodology and Its Application to Nursing, pp. 25-39. New York: John Wiley & Sons, 1981.

Study Activities

1. Describe the three basic principles identified in the Belmont Report.

2. Describe the three requirements in the conduct of research that evolve from the principles.

3. Describe the elements of informed consent.

4. Discuss the three topics related to the protection of human subjects about which the investigator should be concerned and should provide information to the reader.

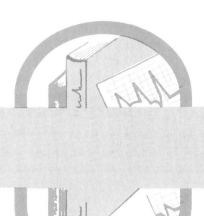

12

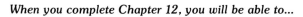

When you complete Chapter 12, you will be able to...

1. Define the functions of the scientific report.

2. Use the analysis questions in the review of research.

QUESTIONS FOR CRITICAL REVIEW

FUNCTIONS OF THE SCIENTIFIC REPORT

A research report is a device for communicating to the scientific community. It should communicate a body of specific data and ideas, detailed enough to permit an informed evaluation. It should be a contribution to the body of scientific knowledge and should stimulate and direct further inquiry (Babbie, 1979). There are many kinds of research reports: short research notes for science bulletins; reports for sponsors; working papers, which are long and tentative; papers delivered at professional meetings; articles published in scientific journals; and books (Babbie, 1979). For our purposes, we are concerned with the critical review of articles published in scientific journals.

The information in the earlier chapters includes some of the rules that must be followed and some of the procedures that must be carried out in order to move from human inquiry to scientific inquiry. Everyone does human inquiry and selects samples and collects data in order to make decisions. The process of collecting information for decision making is common, continuous, and not always conscious; in scientific inquiry, the rules are different, and some of these differences have been described in the preceding chapters.

According to Gay (1976), everyone is a consumer of research, but not a *critical* consumer of research. When the beautiful men and women in the television commercials make their pitch for Brand Best of All, buyers generally do not question control procedures or the appropriateness of inference to people from findings in rats. The public just depends on the findings and goes forth to spend money for the product. Professionals, however, must be able to identify bias and to differentiate good technique from poor technique in research studies. There are responsibilities connected with professionals' work, to be informed concerning the latest findings in their area of expertise and to know enough about each of the components of the research process to be competent evaluators of the soundness of research findings in the profession.

The pressures of professionalism motivate nurses to become informed about research relevant to their practice. The first 11 chapters in this book provide information to help practitioners to do competent evaluation of research findings. All the chapters are instruction chapters, in that they provide information about how, and sometimes why, a necessary task is to be accomplished. Now that you know a little about how research *should* be accomplished, this final instruction chapter is about the procedure of using the information you have acquired in order to carry out critical review of research activities.

Williamson (1981) says that *critiquing* is the thoughtful examination of the research report, consideration of the sources of hypotheses, the study concepts, the appropriateness of the methodology, the validity of the conclusions, and the manner of presenting the study, with the intent of assessing the strengths and weaknesses of the study. The function of a critical review is not to expose all the author's shortcomings. Study merit is as important to the reader as study limitations. The reader needs to know enough about the study to judge its merit and form an opinion of how seriously to take the findings (Polit and Hungler, 1983; Selltiz, Jahoda, Deutsch, and Cook, 1966).

In their discussion of the content of a critique, Brink and Wood (1983) identify three evaluation criteria: usability, completeness, and consistency. Although they are advising investigators concerning the articles that should be included in the literature reviewed for a study, their criteria are also appropriate to the reader, particularly the criteria of usability and consistency.

One component of *usability* is whether the information can be used in practice, and this is a question the clinical utilizer of research must always have answered by a study. *Completeness* is concerned with the ability to replicate the study, and this may not be of immediate interest to the reader, although in a study that can be replicated from the information provided, the author has certainly provided enough information for the reader. *Consistency* is concerned with the logical progress of ideas from the problem through the hypotheses, the data-collection technique, and the analysis and interpretation process. The hypothesis, or the research question, must be derived from the formulation of the problem, and the methodology must provide data clearly relevant to test the hypothesis or answer the research question. Interpretation must tie the findings to the literature described in the formulation of the problem.

The function of a research report is to tell readers about the problem that was investigated, why the problem needed to be investigated, how it was investigated, the results of the investigations, and what the investigator thinks those results mean. Kerlinger (1973) makes a major point about the report of a research study. He says that the function of the investigator is not to *convince* the reader of anything; rather, it is to report concisely and clearly what was done, why it was done, the outcome of the doing, and the conclusions that are drawn from the findings. The report should be written so the reader can come to his own conclusions concerning the strength and accuracy of the findings.

Fox (1969) agrees: he says that the basic function of a research report is to *inform* an audience, and that for information to be communicated, someone must read and understand the report. He points out the importance of the audience of practitioners and says that it is the investigator's responsibility to inform this group of both the results of the research and the implications for practice. He believes that practitioners are necessary to researchers and *vice versa*, and this point is iterated and reiterated in this book.

The research report must inform the reader clearly and completely of the parameters of the problem to be studied, the study process (i.e., the methodology), the results of the analysis, and the investigator's interpretation of the results.

The question now is, how can a clinical practitioner become a critical consumer of research findings? Easy answer: he reads critically. How does he read critically? He follows the critical review process described below by asking a series of questions about the study. Before he does that, however, he assumes an attitude of competence. Remember that it is the responsibility of the writer to write so you can read and understand. If you are really trying and you still cannot figure out what the writer is saying, blame the writer and find another article. This is not to say that the writer is responsible for teaching you simple statistics so you can understand the tables, or sampling techniques, or the necessary steps in the research process; he is responsible for *reporting* these things clearly, using technical language as it is appropriate, but always writing for an audience that speaks English. There is no excuse for obscurity in a research report, and clarity should not be sacrificed to an investigator's urge to write scientific shorthand (Castles, 1975).

Critical review always takes into account the intent of the

investigator. If the design is exploratory, it is proper that the data-collection techniques are flexible and the conclusions tentative and incomplete. If the intent of the investigator is description, the data-collection techniques are expected to provide accurate and comprehensive information, and the investigator must discriminate explicitly between findings applicable only to the sample and findings that may be generalizable to populations. If inferences to populations are made, the range of error must be identified. Explanatory efforts addressing causal relationships require experimental design (Babbie, 1979).

Nobody is perfect, and Brink and Wood (1983) caution us not to throw out the baby with the bathwater. Even a poor research report may have something useful in it, and even the best one will have a flaw or two.

ELEMENTS IN THE DECISION TO READ

With these cautions in mind, how do you begin to read critically? Because the first thing the reader has to do is decide whether or not he wants to read the article, he will start with a set of *decision elements*: these are the *title*, the *author credentials*, the *reference list*, and the *abstract*.

Look at the title. It should give you a clue about what is in the study. A good title includes the major variables to be studied, and maybe even the population that was sampled. It should be long enough to give you some information. In a study about the impact of fear of the environment on nursing performance, in a population of community health nurses, the title should be "The Impact of Environmental Fear on Nursing Performance in Community Health Nurses," not "Fear! Nurses on City Streets!" or something equally exciting and misleading. A good title is informative about the variables of the study.

After you look at the title, you may want to look for author credentials, information concerning the author. Sweeney and Olivieri (1981) suggest educational background and employment site as useful bits of information, and this is provided in many, but not all, journals. You want to know the author's educational background because you will have some questions about a medical doctor writing about nursing interventions, or a sociologist addressing the organizational structure of nursing on a clinical unit, without a coauthor who has nursing credentials. Because nurses know more about nursing variables than anyone else, nursing research is probably best conducted by nurses. You would also like to know if the nurse has a doctoral degree; if he has, you know he has done at least one piece of research under supervision. This is *not* to say that only doctorally prepared nurses can do research, or even that all doctorally prepared nurses can do research, but it is one more clue about the ability of the investigator to investigate. Employment site provides a clue: you would have some questions perhaps about the ability of an investigator employed in an intensive care unit to do a study about the impact of environmental fear on the nursing performance of community health nurses. You would not refuse to read a study on the basis of this kind of information, but you would keep it in mind in case you find something else to question before you get to the study itself.

Sweeney and Olivieri (1981) suggest also a look at the date of publication; if you subtract a year or so (it usually takes a year or more to get a study into print) you will have some useful perspective on the time the study was done, which may help you to understand the interpretation of the data. It is also useful to note the characteristics of the journal in which the research is published: refereed journals, that is, journals in which publication is preceded by review by several experts in the subject of the study, as well as by editorial review, are likely to publish better studies. Such journals have more prestige, as a rule, than do journals in which only editors see the research.

The references should be examined before the decision to read the study is made, to get a sense of their quality as well as the spread of the dates (Sweeney and Olivieri, 1981). Research in nursing is not static, and references should be up to date. As a rule, the majority of the references should be journal articles rather than texts, and they should have publication dates within 5 years or so of the time the study was carried out. Understand that this is not a hard and fast rule; the desired characteristics of the reference section of a report of nursing research are presented in general terms. Sometimes a reference is a classic and must be included in any discussion of certain variables. Sometimes there is little material to be found about a subject, and the author references everything, regardless of its age. Also, because primary sources, documents of the work produced by an author, are to be preferred to secondary sources, documents written about an author's work produced by someone else, some references may be elderly and still be appropriate. For certain kinds of historical research, recency may not be a factor. However, if a clinical research study is published in 1985, and there are no references dated after 1970, you may have the feeling that the literature review is incomplete.

Bear in mind that you, as a reader, are probably also a content expert in the material you are reading, and you may know which authors should be included in the literature review. Certainly nurses working in intensive care units may not know which authors have written about environmental fear in community nursing practice, but they are probably not reading research on this topic. They will be reading about the nursing care of patients on respirators, and they will know who has written about that and who should be included in the investigator's references. The point is, if the investigator has not referenced someone you think should have been included in a review, you can wonder about the findings, and may even wonder about how informed the investigator really is.

Most journals require that an author provide an abstract; this is usually to be found in small print directly under the title and preceding the research report. Sometimes it is even labeled "Abstract." It is there to tell you in 250 to 300 well-chosen words the purpose of the study, the major variables, the population, the data-collection techniques· used, the major statistical findings, and the major conclusions drawn from them. Note the frequent use of the word *major* in this description. It is impossible to tell *all* in 300 words, even if they are well chosen. When there is a good abstract, however, the article itself holds no surprises for the reader, at least no *major* surprises.

The reader may be willing to dispense with investigator conclusions in an abstract, if there is not enough space for everything, but it is useful to know who did what to whom, how, for what reasons, and what the major findings are before beginning the article. An abstract should provide this information.

If there is no abstract, look at the last page of the article for a section called *summary*. This is a brief restatement of the problem, the procedures, the major findings, and the major conclusions (Selltiz et al., 1966). It may function as an abstract for the inquiring reader, in the absence of that useful paragraph at the beginning of the article.

CONTEXT OF THE STUDY

In an article published in an academic journal, there will not be a section called formulation of the problem. There may or may not even be a section called literature review. Both of these steps in the research process are described by investigators in a section that may be called background, or introduction, or relevant literature, or some other such heading. Whatever the section is called, it is placed first in the article, and it presents for a reader's information the investigator's *report* and *interpretation* of the studies he has considered relevant to his study. The interpretation should include many of the factors of the problem that sent him to the literature in the first place, so that the formulation of the problem can be done by the reader on the basis of the concepts and findings in the literature, which are reported by the author. Some of the major factors of the problem are reflected in the literature review, and *all* the concepts or variables described in the statement of the purpose and the hypotheses or research questions should be found there.

The final paragraph in this section should contain the statement of the purpose of the study, the hypotheses to be tested, and/or the research questions to be answered. Sometimes these are provided earlier, but because they should evolve from the problem and the relevant literature, placement at the end of this presentation is appropriate.

Now, as you, the reader, proceed through the background material, which provides the scientific context of the study, to the study purpose and the research questions, what questions do you ask, and how should they be answered? Begin to look for consistency, the logical progress of ideas, from problem to purpose to hypothesis or research question, and into methodology, and analysis and interpretation (Brink and Wood, 1983). The nature of the problem from which the purpose is selected and the nature of the literature about the problem should be clear to you when you get to the statement of the purpose.

Formulation of the Problem

Four major questions can be asked about the formulation of the problem.

1. *Are you able to identify the broad area of interest from which the purpose develops?* Can you formulate the investigator's problem? If he does not do that task for you, explicitly, he should provide you with the information that will allow you to do it for yourself and should do so in the first several paragraphs of the report. Remember that a problem covers a broad domain and is formulated in abstract terms. What *concepts* are being addressed? Selltiz et al. (1966) say that the reader needs to be told enough about the study to place it in a general scientific context.

The context may or may not be theoretical; at the least, the parameters of the problem should be developed in some form of a conceptual framework. The point here is related to the significance, the importance, of the study findings. The investigator who *starts* the study report by saying, "The purpose of this study is to determine the relationship between scores on a satisfaction with nursing scale and opportunity to negotiate care in a population of institutionalized patients" may be telling the reader exactly what the study is about, but what will he do with the findings when he gets them? If he finds that for the 30 subjects in the sample, subjects who were able to negotiate with nurses about care factors were more satisfied than those who were not able to negotiate, who cares? What difference does it make to anyone but the 30 subjects?

Suppose, however, that he starts the report by saying, "Orem's Self-Care Deficit Theory of Nursing is among several theories of nursing with a strong practice orientation, and the constructs relating the agencies of the patient and the nurse are important to clinical practitioners. The idea that the nursing system is activated and developed only in agreement with the patient, when the patient is competent, may be tested empirically in several ways." He continues with a description of Orem's model and mentions the findings of several authors who have used the constructs as a basis for evaluation of practice. Then he tells us the purpose of his study, and when he finds that negotiation is positively related to satisfaction, he can explain the finding in terms of the previously noted theoretical and empirical literature, which suggests that patients should control decisions about their care.

The literature is about the problem concepts; the investigator's hypotheses about the concepts are tested; the findings are explained in terms of what they say about the concepts and how they articulate with the literature. You begin to see why a clear formulation of the problem is so important. Everything follows from that.

2. *Is the problem important?* Even if you can lodge the findings in the literature about the problem concepts, will it make any difference to anybody? To any theory? Importance can be practical—for instance, nurses will do something different with patients, or organizations will make personnel changes—or theoretical—for instance, Orem's formulation of the Conditioning Factors holds in a population of adult surgical patients, which suggests, indirectly, that the relationships postulated by the theory exist.

3. *Are the problem concepts identified in the statement of the purpose researchable?* Can the hypothesis be tested or the research questions be answered in a research design? Some extremely important and interesting concepts do not lend themselves to hypothesis development and testing. Is God good? Is revelation a respectable way of knowing? Can a head of state order activities for the good of the state that she would not countenance as a private person? Is the taking of human life justified for reasons of defense of country, or of self, or of religion? The problem must be one that *can* be investigated, using research design.

4. *Is the context of the problem described so that it is apparent what is included and what is excluded from consideration?* You might think that some things that should be included were not, or that too much was included; the point is that you should be able to tell. Anxiety, for instance, is a broad subject. A problem is supposed to be multifaceted and multivariable, but we must be reasonable. In an ecology in which everything appears to be related to everything else, even a multifaceted, multivariable problem has to be limited. Therefore, you should know from your investigator's first few sentences that the concept "anxiety" that is being examined is out of a certain model of anxiety, considered in certain situations and populations, and that genetic etiology is not addressed in the literature review.

Literature Review

Seven questions important to the critical consideration of the literature are as follows.

1. *Does the literature deal with the problem concepts?* The review should be presented in such a way that the reader begins to have information about the problem and the variables that will be considered in the study. Remember that the literature reported must be relevant to the current study.

2. *Is the literature reviewed, or merely reported?* Are you informed not only about who says what, but also about who is in agreement or disagreement with whom? The investigator should tell you whether the authors who are reviewed had difficulties with their methodologies and whether these difficulties influenced the reliability and the validity of their findings.

3. *Are both theoretical and empirical studies considered?* It is perfectly respectable for the author to do a straightforward, theory-free evaluation, but he must be explicit about what he is doing and must not suddenly include a theory later on to explain the findings. However, if he is testing hypotheses derived from theory, the literature review must include the theoretical material. If the author is doing a study based in a theoretical model, that theory should be described so that you understand the relationships being tested in the study.

In the problem formulated by John Alden in Chapter 4, there is a statement suggesting that the need to identify self-care deficits and establish nursing systems in a population of patients should be independent of medical prognosis. The concepts of self-care deficit and nursing systems are obviously based in Orem's Self-Care Deficit Theory of Nursing. If Alden wants to test the hypothesis that medical prognosis influences nursing care such that fewer self-care deficits are identified in a population of terminal patients than in a population of nonterminal patients, he must describe in his review of the literature the theoretical connections between self-care deficit and the development of nursing systems.

4. *If the author is doing a study with a nontheoretical conceptual framework, are the pertinent concepts and their relationships clearly described?* Even an exploratory study should be organized around some postulated conceptual relationships.

5. *Does the review flow so that the material that is least related to the current study is presented first, with the most relevant material just before the statement of the purpose?* The first few paragraphs of the literature review should present the material that is pertinent in a general way to the concepts of the problem, but not necessarily specific to the current study. The last paragraphs should point specifically to the study purpose.

6. *Is the documentation of the sources clear and complete?*

You should be able to find the references, if you want to do so, from the information given.

7. *Does the investigator conclude the literature section with the implications in the literature, so you know how he got to the hypotheses or research questions?* You should be able to tell from the background material presented the major positions of previous investigators, the findings that are relevant to the current study, and what *your* author thinks of these positions and findings. After you have read the material, you should understand why the investigator has chosen the variables of the study. The references should deal with the study topic or the study methodology and justify the operational definitions of concepts and variables developed by the investigator (Wilson, 1985).

Purpose and Hypotheses

The four questions in this section relate to consistency and to indications of relationships among variables in the statement of the purpose and in the hypotheses.

1. *Does the statement of the purpose clearly derive from the problem concepts and the studies described?* You should understand from the background material presented how the investigator got to the purpose.

2. *Are the major study concepts or variables mentioned in the statement of the purpose?* You may not be able to answer this question until after you have read the methods section, but you should always keep it in mind. Remember, though, that the purpose may mention specific *variables*, or it may not. The purpose is the portion of the problem to be addressed in the study; it may present the *concepts*, rather than the variables that represent the concepts. The purpose may be to test the hypotheses presented later. Sometimes it includes the identification of the population, sometimes not. It should tell you what the study is about, but it may do so in general terms.

3. *Are the hypotheses (or research questions) derived from the purpose?* If the purpose is to test the impact of a specified nursing intervention on anxiety in patients and the hypothesis predicts a relationship between the intervention and patient satisfaction, raise your eyebrows in a superior way and wonder what the investigator can be thinking of.

4. *Are the hypotheses (or research questions) predictions (or questions) about relationships between measurable variables?* At this level, operational definitions are useful. Your investigator is not *required* to indicate in the hypothesis how the variables are measured, but it is not a bad idea. At any rate, the predictions or questions should be about relationships between measurable variables, whether or not the measurements are indicated here. Hypotheses and research questions should be specific enough that you understand what is measured and what concept it represents.

Continue to seek the logical progress of ideas. The problem is broad, significant, conceptual. The purpose is the focus of the current study; it is derived from the problem, may be somewhat general and reflect concepts, or may be more specific and reflect variables. Hypotheses and research questions are narrowly focused and entirely specific, and they consider relationships among measurable variables. The problem may not be fully formulated, but from the background material presented by the investigator, you should be able to name the concepts from which the statement of the purpose and the hypotheses or research questions are derived.

DATA-COLLECTION ACTIVITIES

The research procedures are described in the methods section. The investigator should say how the study was carried out, what the basic design was, and how the instruments were tested for reliability and validity. The population should be identified and the sample-selection process described. If the design was experimental, the investigator should describe the experimental manipulations. If the data collection was by self-report, the kinds of questions that were asked should be noted; the investigator should indicate how the interviewers were trained and how experienced they were. If data collection was by observation, there should be a description of the instructions given to observers and the measures taken to assure reliability and an explanation of how responses are translated into scores. The description of the data-collection process should include who the subjects were, how they were selected from the population, and how they were assigned to treatment groups (Selltiz et al., 1966).

If you have not been informed about this earlier in the report, this is a good place for the investigator to indicate whether or not he is replicating another study and, if he is, what kind of replication it is. He may be doing a direct, literal replication of his own work, in an effort to establish reliability. He may be doing operational replication, that is, trying to duplicate exactly the sampling and experimental procedures used by someone else. Or he may be doing constructive replication, in which he tests findings established by a previous investigator, using his own sampling techniques, data-collection techniques, and analyses. Or he may be doing an entirely new study. In any case, he should let you know which it is, since the fact of replication may explain his selection of subjects and his data-collection techniques.

Subjects

There are six major questions concerned with the population, the sampling procedures, and the protection of the subjects to ask about the subjects in the study.

1. *Is the target population identified?* You should know *from* what group the subjects were selected and *to* what group the investigator plans to generalize the findings. Perhaps it is the entire population that is studied, and generalization of the findings is not an issue. You should not have to make an educated guess about this; the information should be provided.

2. *Are the subjects fully informed about the study and freely consenting volunteers?* There is usually little information about the process of informed consent in research reports; more information should be provided. The investigator should inform you, at the least, that the proposal was reviewed by an Institutional Review Board and that the subjects were volunteers. Of course, if they were not volunteers and deceptive techniques were used, a full description and defense of the deception are required.

3. *How were the subjects chosen to be in the study?* You need enough information about this to be able to identify sources of bias. You would like to see a straightforward statement along the lines of "Subjects were randomly selected from the list of all the patients in the hospital on the 3 days the data were collected." This tells you the target population and that the sample can be considered representative of that population. Whether or not you believe the findings can be generalized to other similar populations—for instance, patients in that hospital on all the other days in the year or patients in hospitals all across the country—may depend on how persuasive the investigator is and how willing you are to accept some logical assumptions about the similarity of one hospital to other hospitals on some characteristics.

If the investigator does not say that the sample was random, you assume that it was not. If the investigator then generalizes the sample findings to the population, you know what you think about that. If the sample is not random, the least the investigator can do is to indicate the likely sources of bias and what that means to the findings. In any case, the sample-selection technique should be made clear and the characteristics of the sample described.

4. *Is the size of the sample adequate?* This usually means are there enough subjects to meet the requirements of the statistics for frequencies in cells, and you may not know that requirement. The investigator worries about size and usually makes some comment about why the size is what it is. In clinical nursing research, the comment is usually something about the fact that the size of the sample limits the generalizability of the study findings. Size is the important information for the critical reader, but the implications of the size for the findings should also be made explicit by the investigator. You should not have to guess about this; the investigator should tell you. You can figure out for yourself that you will not change your nursing care plan on the basis of findings from a study with 10 subjects, even if experimental rigor was maintained; but the investigator should

indicate the impact of a small sample size on the interpretation of the findings.

5. *What was the response rate?* You should be informed how many of the selected subjects actually participated in the study. The investigator probably does not have information about the differences in respondents and nonrespondents that may be relevant to the study variables. If only half the questionnaires distributed were returned, this must be considered in the interpretation of the findings. In a study of patient satisfaction with nursing care, if only half the patients return the satisfaction questionnaire and 10 per cent of them are dissatisfied, is the dissatisfaction ratio 10:100, or is it 10:50? The investigator does not know, and neither do you.

6. *How were subjects assigned to treatment groups?* In an exploratory design, this question will probably not arise; it may be necessary to ask it in a descriptive study. It certainly must be asked in an experimental study that tests causal hypotheses. Remember that, in experimental design, the investigator must be able to carry out random selection of subjects and then randomly assign them to groups. If subjects are assigned to groups on the basis of characteristics that the investigator does not control, he has not protected against unknown sources of bias. Suppose that the experimental group consists of all the patients on the seventh floor and that the control group consists of all the patients on the sixth floor. Maybe the nursing intervention was responsible for the patient outcome, or maybe the patients in the experimental group did better because the seventh floor has many private rooms and wealthier patients are assigned there. A relationship between health and wealth exists in this country, such that the experimental group was probably in better shape to begin with.

Instruments

The data-collection instruments should be appended to the study or described clearly and in some detail. In reports in scientific journals, the complete instrument is usually not provided, since space is at a premium. This is a question of editorial judgment and should not be charged to the author. In the absence of the instrument itself, the author is responsible for giving a fairly detailed description, which will allow you to answer the following seven questions:

1. *Is there still a logical progression of ideas?* The instruments should reflect the problem concepts as these have been presented in the background materials. They should measure the variables and the relationships among the variables presented in the hypotheses or the research questions. It should be clear how they *operationalize* the variables. If the investigator has hypothesized a relationship between level of anxiety preoperatively and the kind of information provided about the postoperative course, the instruments must measure the level of anxiety and describe

the kind of information presented. Remember, there are two kinds of operational definitions: measured operational definitions, which indicate how the dependent variable is measured, the score on the anxiety test; and experimental operational definitions, which indicate how the independent variable is manipulated, the description of the kinds of information provided.

2. *Is the instrumentation appropriate for the subjects and the setting?* Some populations in the health-care setting are vulnerable to fatigue or are easily frightened, or distressed, or coerced. Or the subjects are not in shape to comprehend difficult items, or are uncomfortable being observed. Data collection should be as easy on the subjects as possible. It is hardly appropriate to ask subjects who are institutionalized and elderly to complete a 100-item health-related questionnaire that takes 3 hours to finish and that has many items related to drug use and sexuality. Fatigue and distress will set in fairly early. Along with not being respectful of human needs, such instruments provide biased data, since fatigue and distress contaminate responses in unknown ways. A nurse investigator who wishes to study grief in parents of hospitalized dying children will observe or interview the subjects. She will not send them a questionnaire with 50 open-ended questions requiring several paragraphs of written response, nor will she use the childrens' hospital records as her sole source of information about parental grief.

3. *Were the instruments developed by the investigator or freely adapted from other instruments, or were they standardized tests taken from other studies?* If instruments are original or adapted, full developmental information should be provided. If they are taken *in toto* from others' work, it is still necessary for the investigator to provide the reliability and validity coefficients found by the other authors and to defend their use in a different population.

4. *For original or adapted instruments, how were they developed?* The decision as to what information will be collected and how it will be categorized and scored has to be based on something. Information-seeking items can reflect a theoretical model or a pragmatic conceptual framework. In either case, items should be concerned with study variables. The point is that every information-seeking item on the instrument should make sense in terms of the study concepts. The good investigator knows why he wants the information. He does not ask questions just to be asking, even in exploratory work.

5. *What tests for reliability and validity were made?* The investigator should identify the population in which the instrument was tested. The reader should ask if the tests for reliability and validity are appropriate for the study design. If several raters are using an observation schedule to rate nursing performance, it is not enough to provide an estimate of internal consistency;

interrater reliability must be tested. If theoretical relationships have generated hypotheses, it is not enough to talk about content validity; some effort at establishing construct validity must be made.

New or adapted instruments should be tested in the same populations as the ones from which the study samples will be selected, and the pilot test should be described. Pilot work has two functions: to see if the instrument can be used in the population, for instance, do the subjects understand the items, is the instrument too long; and to develop estimates of reliability and validity. The critical reader asks two questions about the estimates of reliability and validity: Are they the *appropriate* estimates? and Is the magnitude respectable?

Whether the estimates are appropriate depends on what the investigator is trying to do and will vary from study to study. If a new instrument purports to measure a characteristic that can already be measured by a standardized instrument, certainly some form of criterion-oriented validity is indicated, as well as an estimate of equivalence. In studies using a theoretical model, some effort to establish construct validity should be reported. The internal consistency and the stability of an instrument are always of interest.

The time required to do all this and the necessity to establish the set of subjects for the pilot tests without contaminating potential subjects for the study may mean that the reliability and validity of the instrumentation are considered as givens or are dealt with as limitations of the study.

What magnitude you may want to consider respectable in a coefficient depends on whether you think like a psychometrician. Psychometricians like reliability estimates derived from traditional measurement theory to be at least .90, to be useful to people working in test construction. Some sociologists and many nurses carrying out clinical studies will be satisfied, if not happy, with estimates of .70. If the instrument is the only one there is, which is frequently true in the younger sciences, the investigator may simply report the estimates and go on with the study. This behavior should be defended a little, though, so the critical reader will realize that the investigator knows better.

Always ask reliable or valid for what purpose in what population. The investigator must give enough information about the instrument development to allow you to decide if the estimates are respectable enough for how the instrument will be used and how the findings will be interpreted. The reliability and validity of the instruments are factors in the interpretation of the findings.

6. *How are the instruments scored?* The categories of response may be identified on the instrument, so that the subject or the rater need only check a box. Or the investigator may do content analysis on responses to open-ended questions, in order

to develop categories of response. Sooner or later the information obtained with the instrument will surface in numerical form, for statistical analysis. The critical reader must know where the numbers come from.

They are assigned by somebody to the variables that are the indicators of the concepts of interest to the investigator. The assigner, usually the investigator, has to be clear about the rules of assignment.

Scoring may be considered at three levels. On the top level is the concept to be considered: it is abstract, not available to sensory evaluation. The second level consists of the events or behaviors, the variables, that are available to sensory evaluation, that are measurable, and that represent the concept. The bottom level is the number level, the numbers that are used in the measurement activity and that are assumed to represent the concept. The levels can be conceptualized as follows:

SCORING PARADIGM

Level	Content	Defining Characteristic
Concept	Anxiety	Abstract; not measurable
Variable	Behavior	Observable; assumed to indicate anxiety
Symbols of measurement	1 2 3 4 5 6 . . .	Assigned to the behavior as scores; assumed to indicate the amount of behavior present; assumed to indicate the amount of the concept present

The numbers are the scores. They are what will be used in the statistical analysis that provides the findings. The investigator rates the subjects' behavior and says that subjects who score 5 are highly anxious and subjects who score 1 are not anxious. Implicit in this are the assumptions that the behavior reflects the concept and the relations that hold between the numbers on the scale also hold for the behavior and for the concept. The implication is that when a subject scores 3 on the behavior scale, his anxiety level is also 3, and the further assumption is that he is 2 points more anxious than the subject who scored 1 on the activity scale.

Differences in the scores are taken to imply similar differences in the concept. Given all these implicit assumptions about the vertical relationships that hold among the levels, the critical reader should be provided at least with the rationale for the use of a certain kind of scale, a certain technique of scoring.

7. *Do the instruments provide the information necessary to test all the research hypotheses, or to answer all the research questions?* The items should be comprehensive of the hypotheses or the question. If there are two hypotheses, one about level of

stress and one about the etiology of stress, the instrument should provide information about both stress variables.

Application of Instruments to Subjects

After the subjects are selected from the population and the instruments are developed, there is a further set of questions related to how the instruments are applied to the subjects to collect the data. Five such questions are discussed here.

1. *What does the investigator do to the subjects, or what must the subjects do, to provide the information necessary to test the hypotheses or to answer the research questions?* The investigator should provide enough information about the process of using the instruments in the sample that the reader can know what occurred.

2. *In experimental design, how was the independent variable manipulated?* The experimental operational definition should be provided; if the variable is *reinforcement*, and the levels of the variable are *positive notice* and *negative notice*, the techniques of providing positive notice and the techniques of providing negative notice must be spelled out.

3. *How were extraneous variables controlled?* Under laboratory conditions, the question is easily answered, but much health-related research is carried out in field experiments. Certainly studies that address clinical issues are subject to the effect of known and unknown extraneous variables. The investigator depends on random selection and random assignment to groups to control for unknown factors that may influence his dependent variable. Organismic variables, for example, age and gender, and demographic variables, for example, income and education, are controlled by sampling techniques and statistical manipulation. These activities should be reported to the reader.

4. *Will the manipulation and the control procedures test the hypotheses?* No matter how well controlled the experiment is, the experimental activities must test the hypotheses to be useful. The critical reader does not assume that the procedures test the hypothesis, although usually they do; after all, that is the intent of the design. But the reader has his own thoughts about whether there is enough difference in the levels of the experimental variable to make a difference to the dependent variable. For example, in the reinforcement study, is the negative notice *really* negative? In a study of the impact of stress on behavior, is the stress really harsh enough to affect people who know they are in an experiment?

5. *What are the likely sources of bias in the data-collection techniques?* Subjects become fatigued or may be passively resistant. Research assistants also may be fatigued or passively resistant and may not always act according to the research protocol. No matter how reliable and valid the instrument is, the human factor

imposed by the subjects and the data collectors is always a possible source of error.

RESULTS

Authors who write methods texts do not disagree much about the questions a critical reader should ask. They do not use the same language, and some provide a more comprehensive set of questions than others, but all look for pretty much the same things in a research report. The questions in the preceding sections of this chapter are not too different from the questions suggested in other texts, although in this book there is more information about what to look for.

In the results section, the difference between this book and more advanced texts becomes much greater. Those authors who suggest questions about the appropriateness of the statistical tests and the characteristics of the tables are addressing well-informed readers. The position in this book is that you can be a critical reader without being well informed about statistics, and none of the chapters in this book tell you what statistics the investigators should be using.

The results section, therefore, will contain fewer questions for you to consider, not as many as are suggested by other authors. This is not to say that the questions should not be asked. It is to say that you are not likely to know enough to answer them. You must trust the editors not to print studies in which the statistics are not appropriate, or you must ask for advice from someone who can evaluate the statistics used by the investigator.

When it is necessary for you to become well informed enough to deal with the statistical manipulations, you will no longer be using this book. For those of you who do not become so well informed about statistics, there are still a few questions to consider in the investigator's analysis of the data and presentation of the findings.

1. *Does the analysis deal with* all *the information obtained that is relevant to the questions asked or the hypotheses tested?* The investigator cannot choose to ignore evidence that does not support his thesis. He must use everything, and he must report on all the points of the research question/hypotheses, even if all he can say is that the question was not answered or the hypothesis was not tested.

He can also consider new relationships that were not predicted, if he chooses to do so, but the primary task is to analyze the information about the variables he has identified. He can look at his data and choose what is relevant, guided by the formulation of the problem, but if the negative evidence is relevant, it must be reported (Selltiz et al., 1966).

2. *Does the investigator present the rationale for a particular analysis?* You may not understand the rationale for the use of the statistics, and you will take his word that these statistics are appropriate, but the rationale should be there.

3. *Do the findings test the hypotheses or answer the research question?* If the question is whether there is a relationship between gender and levels of aggression, the mean aggression score of a sample of women and the mean aggression score of a sample of men may be obtained; there ought to be a finding in statistical form about whether the two means are different and whether the difference is statistically significant.

All the variables must be considered in the presentation of the results. After findings related to the study variables are presented and discussed, the investigator may present the unexpected findings and talk about them a little. However, the logical progression of ideas requires that the concepts and variables considered in the conceptualization of the study must also be considered in the analysis and interpretation of the data, even if the findings are negative or inconclusive. These variables are what the study was about; if it turns out that the study should have been about something else, they still must be considered.

Sometimes it is necessary to present a rationale for not presenting findings related to the study variables in full. Owing to difficulties like a high attrition rate in the sample or a faulty instrument, information relevant to these variables may not have been obtained, or it may be worthless. There is certainly no reason to use up space reporting findings that have no value, but the explanation should be offered.

4. *Are the categories of response developed correctly?* They should be set up according to the research purpose; be mutually exclusive and independent, exhaustive, derived from one classification principle; and be on one level of discourse. You know the requirements for developing good categories of response. If the categorization was slipshod, the results of the analysis are not valid.

5. *Are the statistical manipulations descriptive or inferential in nature?* If the investigator is simply describing the sample or describing an association between variables, the results are straightforward. However, if inferences are being made about populations from the sample findings, different questions must be asked. The statistics themselves may be the same, but they are used in a different manner. The functions of the statistics should be made clear to the reader.

Babbie (1979) says that the presentation of the data analyses should provide a maximum of detail without being cluttered. He believes that quantitative data presentations should permit recomputations by the reader, although this is no reason for you to panic, since recomputation is not *required* of the reader; there is a school of thought which says it should be possible, though.

INTERPRETATIONS AND IMPLICATIONS

The process of interpretation of the findings and identification of the implications for theory and for practice allows the author some latitude. It is in interpretation that the investigator may be most creative and free wheeling. However, there are still a few questions from the critical reader.

1. *Are all the inferences firmly based in the findings?* If patient satisfaction scores are higher on the Primary Nursing Unit than they are on the Team Nursing Unit, does the investigator suggest that that "means" we should all do primary nursing? Or even that patients like primary nursing better? The investigator would certainly like to say that the difference "means" something more than just a variation in this sample, but he has moved a good distance from the findings when he begins to pontificate about how all nursing should be. On the other hand, if he just reports the difference in the sample and does not attempt to interpret the difference in broader terms, we are back to "who cares?" All the findings must be interpreted, and all the interpretations must be based in the findings. How far you are willing to allow an investigator to go depends, to some extent, on your own comfort with free-wheeling discussion, but the interpretation should always have some logical basis in the findings.

2. *Are the interpretations lodged in the literature?* Remember that the investigator *may* look for the meaning of the findings within the bounds of the study, particularly in evaluation research, when the answer to "who cares?" is "the people who commissioned the study." Usually, however, the investigator is interested in assigning a broader meaning to the findings: the difference in the sample groups indicates a difference in the population groups. Or the difference in the groups on the variable suggests different behaviors in life settings; for example, nurses scoring high on an empathy scale will *behave* in a different manner from nurses scoring low on an empathy scale.

To develop the broader interpretation, the investigator must return to the theoretical and empirical literature with his findings and indicate how they articulate with the theoretical constructs and the results of other studies. The critical reader does not accept the interpretation as a given, but must decide whether the investigator can really attribute all that meaning to the findings. The reader always inquires whether the results are sound and whether the meaning attributed to the results is logical and plausible.

3. *Does the investigator address the implications of his interpretations?* The implications of the knowledge that has been added to the nursing lore should be considered. If the findings are interpreted to support theoretical constructs, the extent and the nature of the support and what it means to the verification of the theory should be discussed.

Explicit implications for the practice of nursing are not to be found in every nursing study and should not be dragged in as a final paragraph because it is fashionable to be interested in contributing to practice. If the investigator expects his findings to have such implications, he should bring it up in the conceptual material, so he can refer to it in his discussion.

USE OF NURSING RESEARCH

There are a final few paragraphs for the nurse who is becoming a critical reader. These are concerned with the relationship between nursing research and nursing practice and with how nursing research is used.

In her report of the Conduct and Utilization of Research in Nursing Project (CURN), Horsley includes a monograph called *Using Research to Improve Nursing Practice: A Guide* (Horsley, Crane, Crabtree, and Wood, 1983). The authors identify the difference in goals of the nurse scientists and the nurse clinicians, the focus on the group versus the focus on the individual. They indicate that the purpose of the monograph is to help nurses to use research as a basis for practice and suggest that research and the use of research are interdependent processes that help to further nursing science. They go so far as to suggest that "together they can be viewed as research activity" (p. 2). They view research utilization as systematic and identify the activities that constitute utilization. These are:

1. The identification and synthesis of multiple research studies in a common conceptual area, which forms the research base.
2. The transformation of knowledge derived from the research base into a solution, or clinical protocol.
3. The transformation of the clinical protocol into specific nursing actions that are administered to patients, the innovations.
4. A clinical evaluation of the new practice to ascertain whether it produced the predicted results (p. 2).

This is an *organizational* activity, since the development of the clinical protocols as these are described in the CURN project requires administrative frameworks as well as clinical expertise. They view research utilization as "an organizational process to be carried out by and for the total nursing staff in a department of nursing" (p. 2). They perceive that the availability of research-based protocols is an essential aspect of the research utilization process. Unfortunately, they are correct.

In the best of all possible worlds, a developing science and a developing practice would proceed in this entirely logical fashion. In the world we live in, to depend entirely on this organizational model would mean that the science and the practice would develop very slowly, if at all.

Not every organization will be amenable to the development and use of the clinical protocols and to the organized departmental research effort. Individual activity can also be useful. If, as Styles (1982) suggests, the development of a profession depends on the development of professional behavior in the individual members, such individual activity is, at best, a strong addition to the organization effort and at worst, is better than nothing.

Clinical nurses who are interested in research in clinical settings would do well to invest in the Horsley et al. guide. Those nursing administrators who are trying to move nursing departments in the direction of research use will certainly find it helpful.

Students of this book are certainly qualified to participate in the effort to bring nursing research to the level of clinical and organizational importance now held by medical research. If the effort is unsuccessful, the critical reader can still use research findings to adapt individual care plans.

References

Babbie, E.R. The Practice of Social Research. 2d ed. Belmont, Calif.: Wadsworth, 1979.

Brink, P.J., and M.J. Wood. Basic Steps in Planning Nursing Research, from Question to Proposal. 2d ed. Monterey, Calif.: Wadsworth, 1983.

Castles, M.R. A practitioner's guide to utilization of research findings. Journal of Obstetrical/Gynecological Nursing, January/February (1975): 50-53.

Fox, D.J. The Research Process in Education. New York: Holt, Rinehart & Winston, 1969.

Gay, L.R. Educational Research: Competencies for Analysis and Application. Columbus, Ohio: Merrill, 1976.

Horsley, J.A., J. Crane, M.K. Crabtree, and D.J. Wood. Using Research to Improve Nursing Practice. New York: Grune & Stratton, 1983.

Kerlinger, F.N. Foundations of Behavioral Research. 2d ed. New York: Holt, Rinehart & Winston, 1973.

Polit, D., and B. Hungler. Nursing Research: Principles and Methods. 2d ed. Philadelphia: J.B. Lippincott, 1983.

Selltiz, C., M. Jahoda, M. Deutsch, and S.W. Cook. Research Methods in Social Relations. New York: Holt, Rinehart & Winston, 1966.

Styles, M. On Nursing: Toward a New Management. St. Louis: C.V. Mosby, 1982.

Sweeney, M.A., and P. Olivieri. An Introduction to Nursing Research: Research, Measurement and Computers in Nursing. Philadelphia: J. B. Lippincott, 1981.

Williamson, Y.M. Critiquing and reporting. In Y.M. Williamson ed. Research Methodology and Its Application to Nursing, pp. 289-299. New York: John Wiley & Sons, 1981.

Wilson, H.S. Research in Nursing. Menlo Park, Calif.: Addison-Wesley, 1985.

APPENDIX

CRITICAL REVIEW
DEMONSTRATED

The article reviewed here is "Environmental Support for Autonomy in the Institutionalized Elderly" by Muriel B. Ryden. It was published in *Research in Nursing and Health* 8:363-371, in 1985, and is reprinted by permission of the publishers, John Wiley & Sons. Dr. Ryden is commended for her willingness to let her work serve in a demonstration project for undergraduate nursing students.

Note that when you are referred in the appendix to page numbers and paragraph numbers, the pages referenced are the original page numbers of the article, reproduced with the article.

Research in Nursing & Health, 1985, 8, 363–371

Environmental Support for Autonomy in the Institutionalized Elderly

Muriel B. Ryden

The climate for autonomy in four urban proprietary nursing homes was investigated as part of a larger study of the relationship between perceived control and morale. Data from 113 residents, 137 caregivers, and 10 administrative personnel revealed that caregivers see themselves as the predominant decision makers. Although they prefer a slightly higher level of self-determination for residents, only in one-to-one and solitary activities do they prefer giving residents the primary decision making role, possibly because they see most residents as not capable of making decisions. Residents saw themselves as having more control than did staff. Grooming and eating were identified by both groups as areas where residents had the least control. A substantial proportion of caregivers and administrative staff did not emphasize the availability of options to residents.

Studies of control and morale among elderly persons have shown a generally consistent, positive relationship between a sense of internal control and various indices of well-being. Descriptive studies by Chang (1978a); Elias, Phillips, and Wright (1980); Hulicka, Morganti, and Cataldo (1975); Morganti, Nehrke, and Hulicka (1980); Noelker and Harel (1978); and Pohl and Fuller (1980); and experimental studies by Langer and Roden (1976); Mercer and Kane (1979); and Schulz (1976) supported the hypothesis that a sense of well-being is associated with the perception of self-determination in older persons. Contradictory findings were reported by Felton and Kahana (1974), who found that positive adjustment in institutionalized elderly was associated with perceptions that staff were in control.

Beliefs about expectancy for control have been studied extensively since Rotter's pioneering research on the locus of control construct (1966). Such beliefs tend to represent a continuum from internal control (events seen as contingent on one's own behavior or relatively permanent characteristics) to external control (events perceived as the result of luck, chance, fate, or powerful others). A generalized locus of control represents a relatively stable personality dimension, whereas situational control is more context specific. Chang's work (1978a) suggested that situational control is more important in affecting morale.

A consideration of situation specific perception of control brings into focus the importance of the environment as a variable which affects autonomy and thus has the potential for influencing morale. The environment as a determinant of behavior was depicted by Lewin (1951) in his equation: $B = f(P \times E)$. Behavior, he contended, is a function of the product of characteristics of the person and the environment. Mischel (1968) asserted that properties of the environment may account for more of the variance in behavior than measures of trait qualities or even biographic and demographic background data.

A long-term care facility is the almost exclusive environment for many residents, and has the potential to exert a powerful influence on perceived control. The term "total institution" was used by Goffman (1961) to describe places of

Dr. Muriel B. Ryden, is associate professor, University of Minnesota, Minneapolis.

This article was received on July 17, 1984, was revised, and on November 28, 1984, was accepted for publication.
Request for reprints should be addressed to Dr. Muriel B. Ryden, 6-101 Unit F, 308 Harvard St S.E., Minneapolis, MN 55455.

residence such as nursing homes where a large number of like-situated individuals, isolated from the wider society, lead an enclosed, formally administered round of life. He described how such institutions ". . .corrupt and defile. . .self-determination, autonomy, and freedom of action" (p. 43).

Long-term care facilities present a threat to self-directed functioning of residents, not only because they are "total institutions," but also because they tend to operate under the medical model that historically emphasizes authoritarian powers. The phrase, "It's the doctor's order. . .," is commonly used to justify the behavior of staff in limiting decision making by residents.

The problem of autonomy in long-term care settings is intensified by the fact that many residents have marked physical and mental impairments (Eustis, Greenberg, & Patten, 1984). Yet for many elderly the facility represents their permanent residence, their *home*, not a hospital. How to help such persons to maintain some sense of control over their daily activities when energy is low, physical dependency is great, and cognitive functioning is compromised is an immense challenge to caregivers.

Environmental characteristics relative to the aged were researched by Moos (1976), who was instrumental in the development of the Multiphasic Environmental Assessment Procedure (Moos & Lemke, 1979). Environments, like people, have unique characteristics. A fit between person and environment was identified as important in the adaptation of the elderly by Lawton (1980), who also explored the relationship between differing residential environments and morale (Lawton, 1970; Lawton & Cohen, 1974).

The study reported here was part of a larger study of the relationship between the perception of situational control and morale (Ryden, 1982, 1984). This phase of the study was an initial exploration of aspects of the nursing home environment which constitute a climate that has the potential for influencing the degree of autonomy of residents. The environment was conceptualized as having three aspects that relate to the autonomy of residents: interpersonal, organizational, and physical. The purpose of the study was to delineate characteristics of these three aspects of the environment, with emphasis on the interpersonal aspect, as a basis for subsequent research. With only four facilities in the sample, a quantitative study of the association between perceived control and environmental factors was not practicable.

METHOD

Sample

Four nursing homes were randomly chosen from proprietary facilities in the Minneapolis area. The target was a random sample of 120 residents, with 15 residents on intermediate care and 15 on skilled care at each of the four facilities. Lack of eligible subjects resulted in a final sample of 113: 54 residents on skilled care and 59 on intermediate care. Criteria for selection included: age 60 and over, intermediate or skilled care status, able to understand English, auditory acuity sufficient to participate in an interview, cognitively competent,[1] and an energy level sufficient to participate in the testing procedure. Of a total of 232 randomly selected residents, 88 (37.9%) were ineligible and 31 (13.3%) refused.

Use of these criteria for selection of subjects meant that the sample represented the most competent nursing home residents. The generalizability of the findings thus is limited, since many institutionalized elderly do not meet all of these criteria.

The investigator sought verbal consent from each resident after carefully explaining what participation would involve, assuring privacy and confidentiality, and explicitly stating the right to refuse. Material in large type that described the study was left with the resident. For the staff sample, all personnel who provided nursing care were invited to participate, including registered nurses, licensed practical nurses, and nursing assistants. This sample consisted of 137 caregivers: 44 of 69 possible licensed nurses (63.8%) and 93 of 233 possible nursing assitants (39.9%) from the four facilities. In addition, the administrator, the director of nursing, and the director of in-service education in each facility were invited to participate. Of the 12 in this targeted sample, 2 did not take part: a director of in-service education who had resigned and a director of nursing who did not return the questionnaire after repeated reminders.

Instruments

Two instruments were administered to residents by personal interview to obtain information about the climate for autonomy. The Residents'

[1]Whenever the investigator had cause to question a resident's competence, the Mental Status Questionnaire (Kahn, Goldfarb, Pollack, & Peck, 1960) was administered. Persons scoring less than 8 were ruled ineligible.

Questionnaire is a semistructured measure with one section on demographic information and another section with questions on the residents' views of policies and practices of the facility and privileges and rights of residents. The Situational Control of Daily Activities Scale (SCDA) is a measure developed by Chang (1978b) to determine residents' perceptions of the source of control in eight situations of daily living: ambulation, dressing, eating, grooming, toileting, group activities, one-to-one activities, and solitary activities. Chang reported test-retest reliability of .96 after 3 months and an intercoder reliability of 1.0 for the overall categorization of responses as self-determined or other-determined, and .98 for the coding reliability of categorization by activity.

Two instruments were used with staff. An investigator-designed Measure of Environmental Support for Autonomy included a section on demographic information, and a section about beliefs and practices of staff and policies and structures of the facility that related to the autonomy of residents. The second instrument was the Staff Version of the Situational Control of Daily Activities Scale (Staff SCDA), a modification of the SCDA Scale used with residents. Staff were asked first to respond in terms of the actual situation that is typical for most residents on the unit where they work, and then to respond again in terms of what they preferred. The same eight areas of daily activities were explored to ascertain who makes the determination as to what residents do.

RESULTS

Characteristics of Subjects

The 113 residents in the study ranged in age from 60 to 94, with a mean age of 80.93. Most had less than a 10th grade education, and the majority were in the lower socioeconomic class according to Hollingshead's Two Factor Index (Hollingshead & Redlich, 1958). Over 74% of residents were female, and the median length of stay was 22 months. The 137 caregivers also were predominantly female (89.8%), with the majority nursing assistants (67.9%). Registered nurses (RNs) made up 16.8% of the sample, and licensed practical nurses, 15.3%. Almost three-fourths of the 23 RNs were employed part time; 69.6% reported they had no gerontological nursing content in their basic educational program, and only 8.7% had had any further educational experience in gerontological nursing beyond in-service education.

Interpersonal Environment

Residents and caregivers were similar in their perceptions about how much power residents had in the facility, with about 60% of each group indicating that residents had about as much power as they should have, and about 30% responding that residents had too little power. In contrast, 70% of the administrative staff indicated that residents had less power than they should have.

When asked, "Do you specifically emphasize the availability of choices or options for residents?" 70% of caregivers and 50% of administrative staff responded affirmatively. This leaves a sizable group who apparently do not emphasize choices. One caregiver wrote, "I don't believe residents should have that much say about their lives being they are confined in a nursing home and have to take their medicine."

Residents were queried as to whether they had ever talked personally with the administrator or director of nurses about anything related to their care or activity. Staff also were asked whether residents talked with the administrator or director of nursing. The responses in Table 1 suggest that while some residents may indeed talk with administrative staff about issues related to their care, they represent a small proportion of the total resident population. Few residents in these facilities had any interaction with the director of nursing. However, they did go to other nurses regarding issues of self-determination. When asked what they would do if they personally wanted an exception to the way things were done, the nurse was identified by more persons than any other

Table 1. Resident Interaction with Administrative Staff

Type of Interaction	Residents N = 113 (%)	Caregivers N = 137 (%)	Adm. Staff N = 10 (%)
Talk with Administrator			
yes	16.8	59.1	90
no	81.4	5.1	10
don't know	1.8	30.7	—
no response	1.8	5.1	—
Talk with Director of Nursing*			
yes	7.1	59.9	100
no	92.0	8.8	—
don't know	—	26.3	—
no response	0.9	5.1	—

*Administrators were not asked this question. All other administrative staff responded "yes."

staff member as the person to whom they would go.

Responses to the Staff SCDA provided additional information about the practices of staff regarding the autonomy of residents. In response to questions about who determined various aspects of the eight daily activities, staff responded on a 4-point scale: 1 (staff), 2 (staff with some resident input), 3 (resident with some staff input), and 4 (resident).

Respondents were asked to answer each question in terms of the actual situation that was typical for most residents, and then in terms of the caregivers' preferences. Responses to the actual situation were assumed to reflect caregivers' perceptions of current practices regarding decision making by residents, and from the preferred responses, inferences were made about caregivers' beliefs and values concerning resident self-determination.

Mean Staff SCDA scores (Table 2) show that caregivers see staff as the prominent decision makers in the actual situation. Dressing, eating, grooming, and toileting all had mean scores under 2, reflecting primarily staff involvement in determination about these activities. Mean scores for ambulation and group activities ranged between 2 and 3, signaling joint control. In one-to-one and solitary activities, residents were seen as decision makers. However, even here, the mean scores were closer to 3, indicating staff input rather than independent determination by residents.

When asked their preference about who should make the determination in the eight areas of daily acvivities, caregivers consistently preferred greater control by residents than was the actual practice (Table 2). Eating was the area with the greatest increase in preferred over actual control. However, even in the preferred mode, only one-to-one and solitary activities had mean scores over 3, with the highest less than 3.6. In the other six areas, preferred mean scores ranged between 2 and 3, reflecting a desire for joint determination. Thus, while caregivers preferred more resident control, they wanted to retain a considerable share in the decision making about daily activities. Mean scores of registered nurses, licensed practical nurses, and nursing assistants did not differ significantly in either actual or preferred determination.

Caregivers who worked on intermediate care ascribed a higher level of control to residents than caregivers who worked on skilled care. However, staff who worked with residents at both levels of care had lower mean actual and lower mean preferred scores than those who worked exclusively on skilled care.

The SCDA scale for residents had a simpler format, with each response scored as "self" or "other." If any one of the eight areas was found to have an equal number of "self" and "other" responses, it was categorized as "joint" area of determination. To facilitate comparison with resident responses, a determination was made of what percentage of caregivers perceived that decisions about the actual situation were made by resident, made jointly, or made by staff (Table 3). A score on the Staff SCDA of 1–2 was categorized as "staff," over 2 but less than 3 "joint," and 3–4 "resident."

Although it is interesting to examine caregivers' responses to the Staff SCDA along side residents' responses to the same areas of daily activities, direct comparisons are not justified. Caregivers were responding in terms of what was typical for most residents, not in terms of the cognitively intact residents who comprised the subjects in the study. However, it is noteworthy that grooming and eating were identified by both residents and staff as the areas where residents had the least control. One-to-one and solitary activities were the areas where both groups saw caregivers as having the least control.

Staff varied in their perceptions about the capability of residents to make decisions about their daily activities and care. Over 43% of caregivers and 60% of administrative staff viewed the majority of residents as not capable of making such decisions (Table 4).

Organizational Environment

Characteristics of the organizational environment that may enhance autonomy include mechanisms for enabling residents to exercise their

Table 2. Caregivers' Mean SCDA Scores for Eight Daily Activities (N = 137)

Activity	Actual Score		Preferred Score	
	Mean	SD	Mean	SD
Ambulation	2.001	.651	2.732	.586
Dressing	1.870	.651	2.658	.664
Eating	1.660	.576	2.632	.668
Grooming	1.585	.544	2.366	.723
Toileting	1.806	.645	2.425	.671
Group	2.314	.891	2.974	.738
One-to-One	3.184	.813	3.501	.621
Solitary	3.248	.729	3.572	.491

Table 3. Percentage of Residents and Caregivers Perceiving Resident, Staff, or Joint Situational Control of Eight Daily Activities (N = 113 Residents; 137 Caregivers)

| | Type of Control | | |
Activity	Resident (%)	Joint (%)	Staff (%)
Ambulation			
Residents	83.2	4.4	13.3
Caregivers	10.9	27.0	62.0
Dressing			
Residents	89.4	3.5	7.1
Caregivers	8.8	18.2	73.0
Eating			
Residents	55.8	6.2	38.1
Caregivers	2.2	19.7	78.1
Grooming			
Residents	51.3	26.5	22.1
Caregivers	2.9	13.1	83.9
Toileting			
Residents	92.9	—	7.1
Caregivers	8.8	16.1	75.2
Group			
Residents	93.8	1.8	4.4
Caregivers	35.8	10.2	54.0
One-to-One			
Residents	92.9	5.3	1.8
Caregivers	72.3	10.9	16.8
Solitary			
Residents	96.5	0.9	2.7
Caregivers	100.0	—	—

Table 4. Percentage of Residents Perceived by Staff as Able to Make Decisions about Some Aspects of Their Daily Care

Percentage of Capable Residents	Caregivers (N = 137) (%)	Administrative Staff (N = 10) (%)
75–100	12.4	20
50– 74	43.8	20
25– 49	31.4	60
0– 24	11.7	—

rights, the presence and functions of a Residents' Council, the establishment of a clearly defined grievance process, participation of residents in care planning, the provision of alternative times and menu items for meals, the membership of residents on committees, participation by residents in the publication of newsletters, and policies that enable residents to control their personal allowance, retain items of their own furniture in their rooms, and determine when they leave and return to the nursing home.

All four of the nursing homes studied had established Residents' Councils which met regularly. Despite the fact that meetings were publicized by posting notices, indicating meeting times on activity calendars and newsletters, and announcing the meeting over the loudspeaker, 26.5% of residents were not aware of the existence of the council. Only 27.4% of residents indicated

they had ever brought any concern to a council meeting or to an officer. Some said they had no concerns that needed attention. A number expressed the feeling that it was useless to do so. "Nothing seems to get done," is the way one resident put it. Some persons expressed fear of jeopardizing their stay. Others felt inadequate in stating their concerns. A few voiced negative feelings about the council: "They stir up trouble."

The councils appeared to involve only a small percentage of those who potentially might take part. At the one council meeting at each facility observed by the investigator, attendance ranged from 12 to 29 persons (7%-25% of residents). This level of attendance was typical of the usual pattern, according to Council officers and staff.

When questioned as to the usefulness of the Council, residents' positive responses outweighed the negatives. It was the expressive functions they identified as valuable, however, rather than seeing the council as instrumental in policy formation and decision making.

Although nominally residents were officers of the councils, staff members actually dominated the meetings in three out of four facilities. Administrators gave high rankings to "providing residents with a voice in decision making," which was one among a list of possible purposes for a Residents' Council, but only one administrator reported a consistent pattern of operationalizing that purpose by discussing proposed new or revised policies with the council before implementation.

Minnesota statutes mandate that individuals must be informed of their rights as residents, and that the list of rights must be posted in long-term care facilities. Each facility displayed the Resident's Bill of Rights near the front entrance, and staff reported that a copy was routinely given to residents and families on admission. When asked,

"Are you aware of your rights as a resident?" 49.6% responded affirmatively. Rights seemed unimportant to some. "They always treat me so nice," one responded. Another said, "I don't figure I have rights. I'm glad to have a place to live." The importance of resident rights to one individual was apparent when she pulled out a dog-eared underlined copy and described how she had lodged an official complaint againt the facility.

All four nursing homes had an established grievance process, but this was not well understood. Only 15% of residents were aware of its existence. When caregivers were asked if the facility had an established grievance process, 32.8% said they did not know, 11.7% said no, and 53.3% said yes.

Residents were queried as to their access to information by the question, "How do you find out about new policies and regulations that affect you?" Over half of the residents were able to identify some source of information, including staff, the newsletter, meetings, and other residents. However, 21.2% were uncertain, and 19.5% did not respond. A few (5.3%) indicated that they were kept in the dark. "They don't communicate. They keep things quiet," said one. Another said, "I don't think they let me know anything." When asked, "Do you take part when staff review your care plan?" 56.7% said they did not, 8.8% said they did take part, and 4.5% did not know. A greater degree of involvement was seen in responses to the questions, "If a new medicine or treatment is proposed for your care by the doctor or nurse, do you have some say in the matter?" Over 42% responded affirmatively, but almost as many (40.7%) said they did not have any input.

Residents were members of established committees in two facilities. These committees dealt with safety, environmental planning, and selection of the employee of the month.

Physical Environment

Findings of the study suggested characteristics of the physical environment that are relevant to the autonomy of residents. One of the most apparent was the limited amount of personal space some residents had. Privacy was a rare commodity, with less than 4% of residents having a private room, 54.9% in double units, 40.7% in triple units, and 1 in a quadruple unit. In some units, beds were placed so close together that there was no more than a width of a bedside stand between them. Negotiating such narrow passages with a wheelchair or walker would challenge an agile, healthy person, and was a real obstacle to persons with visual and motor problems. Such an environment provided a constant barrier to autonomous functioning.

Nevertheless, most residents (68.2%) saw themselves as having either complete control or considerable control over this personal space, no matter how limited. However, 17.7% believed they had little or no control. Staff saw them as having less control over this space. Comments of many residents suggested that their sense of control was related to the behavior of other residents, often a roommate. Friction over ventilation, lighting, and use of radio and television were cited as limitations to control. Only one of the facilities had a designated "Privacy Room" that was available for residents to use. In the others, only 37.2% of residents indicated that a place was available if they wanted privacy for some reason. Lack of privacy also was apparent in the use of telephones. Although 23% of had their own telephones, a substantial proportion (32.7%) said that they could not make a telephone call in private.

Unsolicited comments by residents during the interview revealed another area where the sense of autonomy was threatened. A theme repeated over and over was concern about theft. The physical environment was not structured so as to provide a secure but accessible place for personal belongings. One facility had a locked drawer, but things were not secure there since someone could gain access to the contents by removing the drawers in an adjacent room that were behind the locked drawer.

DISCUSSION

A significant aspect of a climate for autonomy is the atmosphere created by the interactions of staff with residents. Caregivers, more than any other persons, provide the immediate interpersonal environment for institutionalized elderly. They have the opportunity to influence both the objective extent of self-determination and also the resident's subjective sense of situational control. A step further removed from the residents, the administrative staff represent an important power holding group within the facility. While they have less direct interpersonal interaction with residents than do the caregivers, their leadership and teaching functions give them the potential for exerting a broad influence on the interpersonal environment which residents experience.

The finding that a sizable group of administrative staff and caregivers acknowledge that they do not emphasize the availability of choices or options for residents is particularly relevant in light of the experimental studies of Langer and Rodin (1976) and Mercer and Kane (1979), which suggest the impact on morale of explicit emphasis on the availability of choices. This finding may reflect a need for information on the part of administrative staff and caregivers regarding research findings that link perceived control with morale.

Identification of grooming and eating by both residents and staff as areas where residents exerted the least self-determination gives some specific direction to attempts to raise morale by increasing perceived control. Targeting interventions in these two areas might be more productive in increasing a sense of autonomy in residents than experimental manipulations in other areas.

What accounts for the fact that the practice of caregivers as well as their preference regarding control, as evidenced by these data, tend to be so strongly in the direction of staff determination rather than resident self-determination? One of the most likely explanations is the view of many caregivers that residents have only limited capability for decision making (Table 4).

Staff were asked, "What proportion of residents in your facility do you think have the ability to make decisions about some aspects of their daily activities and care?" The capacity to make complex judgments was not the issue posed, but simply the capability to make decisions about some aspects of their daily activities and care. Although caregivers tended to see more residents as capable than did administrators, over 43% believed that less than half of residents had such capabilities. The reality that the nursing home population is indeed comprised of an increasing number of severely mentally impaired residents means that this perception is consistently reinforced, and probably contributes to care givers attributing incompetence to many residents who in fact have the capacity for making many decisions about daily activities. The tendency to generalize may cause staff to conclude that because a resident evidences a specific cognitive impairment such as some memory loss or some degree of disorientation, that he or she is incapable of making decisions about any aspect of daily life.

Support of this hypothesis is suggested by the finding that staff who cared for residents on both skilled and intermediate care had lower actual and preferred scores on the Staff SCDA than those caring for either group exclusively. Perhaps working with residents of varying capacities for decision making contributes to difficulty in individualizing care. Reduced expectations of residents are likely to lead staff to act on behalf of residents when self-determination is possible. The relationship between beliefs about resident competency and the nature of staff-resident interactions regarding decision making needs to be systematically explored.

The fact that many nursing home residents demonstrate some degree of confused behavior is clearly an issue in the practices and preferences of staff that relate to the autonomy of residents. Certainly mental status affects the nature of self-governing behavior. Is a given individual capable of making and communicating any decisions? If so, what kind? What are the risks of specific acts of self-determination? How do such risks compare with the risks of feeling powerless? If memory loss and diminished judgment limit self-control in certain areas, in what other areas may personal control be exerted? Under what conditions does the opportunity to choose and decide cause undue stress? Systematic exploration is needed to answer such questions and to determine how mental status influences the well-documented relationship between a sense of autonomy and a sense of well-being.

The passivity and conformity of many residents may also serve to reinforce caregivers' perceptions regarding the desirability of staff control. The extent to which such passive, conforming behavior is a response to institutionalization or a personality characteristic of those residents that existed prior to admission to a long-term care facility is another interesting question worth investigating.

Another influencing factor may be the desire for control on the part of caregivers. Nursing homes tend to function with a medical model of fairly rigid hierarchical structure. Residents may be viewed by some as being at the bottom of the pecking order. Caregivers, particularly nursing assistants, often experience little control over their work situation except in their interaction with residents. Many nurses have been socialized to control, to take care of, to do for patients.

Yet another factor may be the lack of a knowledge base in gerontology that might provide insight regarding the effects of powerlessness on the aged. Nursing assistants, who represent the bulk of the caregivers, have minimal preparation for providing nursing care to the elderly. Most RNs did not have specific gerontological content in their nursing program, and few had further education in gerontology beyond what had been provided as inservice education.

CRITICAL REVIEW DEMONSTRATED

A commitment to autonomy for residents can be operationalized within the organizational structure of a long-term care facility. Findings of this study suggest that a Resident's Bill of Rights, a formalized grievance process, and a Residents' Council provide potential mechanisms for autonomy. However, at present that potential is far from being realized. Knowledge is power. Despite the availability of information, the extent of the lack of knowledge about these mechanisms among this most competent group of residents limits the extent to which self-determination might exist within the facility. This seems to reflect a need for more individualized efforts at consciousness raising, particularly in view of the visual and auditory impairments of many residents, which restrict their ability to get information from such traditional sources as bulletin boards and loudspeakers. Such efforts cannot take place, however, unless caregivers are themselves informed about mechanisms for self-determination and unless they value autonomous behavior on the part of residents.

The inclusion of residents in a formalized process of care planning to the extent possible can be encouraged by organizational policies. It is not just the big decisions such as orders regarding resuscitation where resident involvement is justified. It is the lack of control over the myriad of everyday activities that can lead to a demoralizing sense of powerlessness (Chang, 1978a; Pohl & Fuller, 1980; Ryden, 1984).

According to Youker (1980), quality of life for nursing home residents can be improved more by increasing the flexibility of nursing home policies and practices than by increasing financial outlays.

As new homes are built and existing facilities updated, planners have the option of constructing physical environments that enhances the self-determining behaviors of residents. The inclusion of representative residents in groups responsible for such planning is a place to start. Efforts to secure access for the handicapped point to many desirable architectural modifications that can be made. Other elements that may encourage autonomous behavior in the elderly were identified in this study.

In conclusion, given research findings that support a positive association between a sense of control and a sense of well being in the aged, efforts to provide a climate for self-determination seem warranted. The findings of this initial exploration of environmental supports for autonomy suggest areas profitable for further investigation.

REFERENCES

Chang, B. L. (1978a). Generalized expectancy, situational perception of control and morale among institutionalized aged. *Nursing Research, 27,* 316–324.

Chang, B. L. (1978b). Perceived situational control of daily activities: A new tool. *Research in Nursing & Health, 1,* 181–188.

Elias, J. W., Phillips, M. E., & Wright, L. L. (1980). Relationship of perceived latitude of choice to morale in a nursing home environment. *Experimental Aging Research, 4,* 357–365.

Eustic, N., Greenberg, J., & Patten, J. (1984). *Long-term care for older persons: A policy perspective.* Monterey, CA: Brooks/Cole.

Felton, B., & Kahana, E. (1974). Adjustment and situationally-bound locus of control among institutionalized aged. *Journal of Gerontology, 29,* 295–301.

Goffman, E. (1961). *Asylums.* Garden City, NY: Anchor Books, Doubleday.

Hollingshead, A. B., & Redlich, F. C. (1958). *Social class and mental illness.* New York: Wiley.

Hulicka, I., Morganti, J. B., & Cataldo, J. (1975). Perceived latitude of choice of institutionalized and noninstitutionalized elderly. *Experimental Aging Research, 1,* 27–39.

Kahn, R. L., Goldfarb, A. I., Pollack, M., & Peck, A. (1960). Brief objective measures for the determination of mental status in the aged. *American Journal of Psychiatry, 117,* 326–328.

Langer, E., & Rodin, J. (1976). The effects of choice and enhanced personal responsibility for the aged. A field experiment in an institutional setting. *Journal of Personal and Social Psychology, 34,* 191–198.

Lawton, M. P. (1970). Assessment, integration and environments for the elderly. *Gerontologist, 10,* 38–46.

Lawton, M. P. (1980). *Environment and aging.* Monterey, CA: Brooks/Cole.

Lawton, M. P., & Cohen, J. (1974). The generality of housing impact on the well-being of older people. *Journal of Gerontology, 29,* 194–204.

Lewin, K. (1951). *Field theory in social science.* New York: Harper & Row.

Mercer, S., & Kane, R. A. (1979). Helplessness and hopelessness among the institutionalized aged: An experiment. *Health and Social Work, 4,* 91–116.

Mischel, W. (1968). *Personality and assessment.* New York: Wiley.

Moos, R. H. (1976). *The human context: Environmental determinants of behavior.* New York: Wiley-Interscience.

Moos, R. H., & Lemke, S. (1979). *Multiphasic environmental assessment procedure: Preliminary manual.* Palo Alto, CA: Social Ecology Laboratory, Stanford University School of Medicine.

Morganti, J., Nehrke, M., & Hulicka, I. (1980). Resident and staff perceptions of latitude of choice

ized men. *Experimental Ag-*
-385.

1978). Predictors of well-
...ong institutionalized aged.
....., *18*, 562–567.

...n, J., & Fuller, S. (1980). Perceived choice, social
interaction, and dimensions of morale of residents in a home for the aged. *Research in Nursing
& Health, 3*, 147–157.

Rotter, J. B. (1966). Generalized expectancies for
internal versus external control of reinforcement.
Psychological Monographs, 80.

Ryden, M. B. (1982). *Perception of situational control,*

*climate for autonomy and morale in institutionalized
elderly.* Unpublished doctoral dissertation, Univ-
erity of Minnesota, Minneapolis.

Ryden, M. B. (1984). Morale and perceived control
in institutionalized elderly. *Nursing Research, 33,*
130–136.

Schultz, R. J. (1976). Effect of control and predictability on physical and psychological well-being
of the institutionalized aged. *Journal of Personality
and Social Psychology, 33,* 563–573.

Youker, P. (1980). *Studies of nursing home care.* Unpublished doctoral dissertation, Florence Heller
Graduate School, Brandeis University, Boston.

DECISION ELEMENTS

Title

The title is informative about the content of the article. Because only one variable is identified (environmental support for autonomy), along with a population (institutionalized elderly), it is clear that the author is not testing causal hypotheses about relationships between variables. On the basis of the title, it is expected that the work is exploratory or descriptive, and this expectation is met.

Author Credentials

The journal is not informative about author credentials, and it is not clear whether the author is a nurse, a sociologist, or both. However, enough information is given for the reader to contact the author if she wants to. The doctoral degree suggests research experience. The employment site is provided but is irrelevant to this study, since the study could be carried out by an academic investigator, or an investigator employed in a service setting.

References

The title suggests that the references should address concepts of control, of autonomy, of environmental influence on self-determination; further, these concepts are considered in a popu-lation that is aged and institutionalized. All of these concepts are found in the reference section. The ratio of books to journals is high, and on first reading, the references are elderly for a study in which, based on the date of the author's dissertation, data were probably collected in 1981-1982. On a closer look, however, the preponderance of non-journal references, as well as the age of many of the references, is explained by the fact that the author has sought primary sources (e.g., Goffman, 1961; Lewin, 1951; Kahn et al., 1960; Rotter, 1966; Hollingshead and Redlich, 1958; and the Moos work, 1976-1979). The journal references are to respectable publications, and the titles suggest that the articles and books have content relevant to the study.

Abstract

The abstract provides enough information for the decision whether or not to read the article to be made. *Research in Nursing and Health* is a refereed journal, so you know that content experts, as well as editors, have reviewed the article. The purpose of the study, investigation of the climate for autonomy in nursing homes, is stated in the abstract, which also describes the samples (residents, caregivers, and administrative personnel), and allows the inference that the target populations are the residents and caregivers in the four nursing homes examined. Sample sizes are given, and major findings are provided. Relevant variables (status and perceived source of control) can be inferred from the findings reported (residents differ from caregivers as to perception of amount of resident control). Explicit identification of the variables addressed would have been useful, but on the whole, the abstract is informative about the major components of the study.

CONTEXT OF THE STUDY

Formulation of the Problem

1. *Can the broad area of interest from which the purpose develops be identified?* Yes. The concepts of control, and its impact on morale, and the impact of environment on behavior are presented in the first few paragraphs, and both empirical and conceptual work is referenced. It is clear that the problem will be formulated around concepts of self-determination as these are affected by an institutional environment for the aged: the concept of morale is not identified in the title or the abstract but may be useful in interpreting the findings and evaluating the significance of the study. No theoretical framework is identified, and none is required in an exploratory study. Lewin's behavior/environment model is mentioned but not in enough detail to suggest that it will be tested. The abstract has indicated that this work is exploratory; the assumption is that the model is accepted as an explanatory device, rather than tested.

It is evident that the broad area of interest is the barriers to self-determination in institutionalized elderly patients. The nursing implications are clear in paragraphs 2 and 3, on page 364; they address the use of the medical model in nursing home care and the characteristics of the residents that sometimes lead caregivers into inappropriate decision making.

The purpose is explicit: it is stated at the end of the background material and derives from that material.

2. *Is the problem important?* Yes. The problem as presented here is important to nursing practice rather than to testing any theory of behavior, or of organization, or of nursing. From the statement of the purpose, one can see that the expectations of the author are tied to subsequent research, which may be theory testing in nature. However, the identification and description of aspects of the environment that may affect self-determination in elderly patients is of importance to nursing in and of itself. Although the study is exploratory and the findings may not be generalizable, they should certainly be suggestive.

3. *Are the problem concepts identified in the statement of the purpose researchable?* Yes. The author does not purport to test relationships between perceived control and the environmental factors (p. 364). No hypotheses or research questions are provided, but the delineation of specified characteristics of the environment (the purpose of the study) can be done using the steps in the research process. Actually, the research questions could have been asked: the report in the abstract of findings concerning the association between status (resident, caregiver) and perception of resident control certainly suggests that the investigator was interested in these relationships. The questions would have provided useful direction to the consideration of the instruments and the sample.

4. *Is the context of the problem described so that it is apparent what is included and what is excluded from consideration?* Yes. It is apparent what is included in this study: "exploration of aspects of the nursing home environment which constitute a climate that has the potential for influencing the degree of autonomy of residents" (p. 364). How the three aspects of the environment to be considered (interpersonal, organizational, physical) constitute the "climate," in some additive or interactional way, is not clear. The exploratory intent of the author is explicit, however, so that full description of the derivation of the concepts is not required, and further explication may wait on further development.

Literature Review

1. *Does the literature deal with the problem concepts?* Yes, to an extent. It deals partly with concepts that may be found in the larger study (the impact of control on morale) but not in this one. Morale is not a variable for this study, which is concerned with the aspects of the environment affecting the autonomy of residents in nursing homes.

2. *Is the literature reviewed, or merely reported?* The literature is reported. Findings are mentioned and conflicts identified (p. 363, the contradictory findings of Felton and Kahana, as

compared with the majority of the authors cited). The conflict is of importance to this study, since it is concerned with relationships between well-being and self-determination in elderly institutionalized subjects. The author does not indicate a reason for the conflict (differences in or problems with methodology? differences in populations?) nor does she identify the set of findings that she believes are the most persuasive. Therefore, her reader knows only that investigators differ on a point of some importance to the present study. None of the studies is evaluated, and in the Goffman work at least, there may be some question as to the impact of passion on cognition. The author describes the variables studied and presents the various findings but does not evaluate or interpret the studies. They are simply presented.

3. *Are both theoretical and empirical studies considered?* To some extent, yes. Both Rotter and Lewin were developing theoretical constructs in their work, and although those models are not used in the development of Ryden's study, they are relevant to the significance of the work. The empirical studies are concerned with the importance of the environment to decision making, adaptation, and morale, and one set of empirical studies provides instruments for this study (Chang). The literature related to the conceptualization of the environment, as this is described in the purpose of the study, is not so clearly in place. Exploratory work may be theory-free, but it would be useful to the reader to know the source of the conceptualization of the environment as having three aspects that relate to the autonomy of the residents (p. 364).

4. *If the author is doing a study with a nontheoretical conceptual framework, are the pertinent concepts and their relationships clearly described?* Not in the section preceding the statement of the purpose of the study. The descriptions emerge in the sections on instruments and results, and the aspects of the environment being explored are addressed in terms of the responses on the instruments. Autonomy is defined implicitly in discussion of the scoring technique (p. 366).

5. *Does the review flow so that the material least related to the current study is presented first, with the most relevant material just before the statement of the purpose?* Yes. The author's perception of the threat to autonomy in the "medical model" operation of long-term care facilities, the physical and mental impairments characteristic of many of the residents, as described by Lawton, and the environmental characteristics explored by Moos are most significant for this study and appear just before the stated purpose.

6. *Is the documentation of the sources clear and complete?* Yes. Comprehensive references are provided, and there are no literature-independent author assumptions to be evaluated. The author stays with her sources in the study design.

7. *Does the investigator conclude the literature section with the implications of the literature, so that the reader knows how the hypothesis or the research question was generated?* The author does not deal with the implications of the literature, and the reader must assume that the findings of the previous studies are acceptable. The purpose of the study is based in the literature.

There is a major strength and a major weakness in the presentation of the background material. The strength is the logical progression of ideas; the purpose (the delineation of characteristics of the environment affecting autonomy) is derived from the larger problem (the impact of perceived control on well-being, morale) *if* the studies describing the impact of environmental variables on perceived control and the impact of control on well-being are acceptable. In this reading, knowledge of the environmental factors affecting autonomy is a precursor to exploring the effects of autonomy on control. The weakness is the lack of evaluation of the studies; the findings are simply presented, with no interpretation from the author and no summary of their implications for the present study.

Purposes and Hypotheses

1. *Does the statement of the purpose clearly derive from the problem concepts and the studies described?* Not entirely. It is not clear that the conceptualization of the environment (interpersonal, organizational, and physical aspects, p. 364) is derived from the literature presented, although the aspects are entirely plausible and the literature is consistent with the instrumentation.

2. *Are the major study concepts or variables mentioned in the statement of the purpose?* The aspects of the environment are identified; there is nothing in the purpose to suggest that residents and caregivers will be compared on their perceptions of autonomy, although the information is provided in the abstract.

3. *Are the hypotheses (or research questions) derived from the purpose?* No hypotheses or research questions are presented. In an exploratory study, these may not be necessary, and the variables *are* developed and operationally defined in the instrument and results sections. Research questions are certainly implicit in the comparisons between groups and the stratification of the residents by skilled- and intermediate-care values, and they would have been useful to the reader. The data collection and analysis activities suggest that the (implicit) questions are derived from the purpose. The purpose is concerned with identifying aspects of the environment that may affect perceived autonomy: the comparisons suggest questions about relationships with status of respondents on all three aspects, since caregivers and residents differ in their perceptions of resident autonomy and of how autonomy is affected by physical and organizational factors.

4. *Are the hypotheses or research questions predictions or questions about relationships between measurable variables?* Not applicable, since no hypotheses are made and the research questions are implicit and not asked here. When the variables are considered in the instrument and results sections, the operational definitions are in place and are consistent with the purpose.

DATA-COLLECTION ACTIVITIES

Subjects

1. *Is the target population identified?* Yes. One set of subjects, the residents, was randomly selected from the population of residents of four nursing homes in a specified area. Criteria of care level, cognition, age, and English-language proficiency required by the study methodology and the author's intent were reported. A second set of subjects, the staff, consisted of volunteers from the population of nursing personnel in the four institutions, all of whom were invited to participate. A third set of subjects was composed of specified nursing and hospital administrators. In all cases it is clear which populations provided the samples. Because only one sample was randomly selected and no treatments are involved, it is equally clear to what populations sample findings may be generalized. In this study, generalization is not an intent of the investigator, and she recognizes the qualities in her sample that make it limited.

2. *Are the subjects fully informed about the study, and freely consenting volunteers?* The author provides good information about how consent to participate was obtained from residents and what information concerning their rights was provided. She indicates how competence to decide is established, and the fact that a description of the study in large type was left with the residents suggests that she did not pressure anyone to sign in a hurry. She has obviously recognized the vulnerability of the population of residents and acted appropriately to protect their rights.

There is less information about the protection of the rights of the nurses and the administrators. The response rates suggest that the members of the most vulnerable nursing group, the nursing assistants, were least likely to volunteer to be in the study. Although they made up the largest portion of the nursing sample (67.9 per cent) because of their numbers in the nursing population, only 39.9 per cent of them volunteered, as compared with 63.8 per cent of the licensed nurses. The purposive sample of administrators is probably not in need of much protection from the investigator, but the size of the sample inhibits anonymity, and this should be addressed.

3. *How were the subjects chosen to be in the study?* The author states that the target was a random sample of 120 residents, equally distributed across care facilities and care levels. The final sample is not that large and the distribution is not equal, but she indicates that random selection continued. From the randomly selected residents, some did not meet the criteria and some would not volunteer. All of the nursing staff in the four groups were invited to participate, and the specified administrators. She has a random sample of residents who volunteered, an accidental sample of an invited population of nurses, and a purposive sample of administrators. The selection technique in each population is clear. Biases related to the fact that all subjects are volunteers are particularly problematic in the sample of nurses. However, the exploratory nature of the study suggests that at this stage, the biases have less importance than they will have later. The demographic characteristics of the resident sample and the nurse sample are described.

4. *Is the size of the sample adequate?* Yes. The data are presented both as mean scores and as percentages; two of the three samples are large enough (more than 100 respondents) to make the use of percentages appropriate, and the means are not subjected to further statistical analysis. The author reports both N and standard deviations with her means, which is commendable.

5. *What was the response rate?* This information is provided for all three groups. Of the 144 eligible residents, 31 refused to participate in the study. When the refusal took place (for instance, before or after the interview) and the reasons for refusal would be useful information in this exploratory study. Some information about how the refusers did or did not differ from the volunteers would also be useful. Certainly the reasons for refusal to participate of 140 of the 233 nursing assistants would be interesting. Reasons are given for the two of the twelve chosen administrators who did not provide data.

6. *How were subjects assigned to treatment groups?* This question is not applicable in an exploratory design.

Instruments

1. *Is there still a logical progression of ideas?* Yes. The instruments as described measure the interpersonal, organizational, and physical aspects of the environment. The interpersonal aspects are addressed in the Situational Control of Daily Activities Scale (SCDA) completed by residents and in the staff version of the SCDA completed by nursing personnel and administrators. The organizational aspect is addressed in the section of the Resident Questionnaire obtaining information about the policies and practices of the institution and the rights of residents, and with the Measure of Environmental Support for Autonomy completed by staff.

It is not clear whether the physical aspects of the environment were measured by these instruments or by an observation schedule (p. 368) that is not described here, but the instruments obviously reflect the problem concepts as these were presented in the background material.

2. *Is the instrumentation appropriate for the subjects and the setting?* The use of interview rather than subject completion of an instrument is appropriate for the most vulnerable of the sets of subjects, the residents, and the items on the SCDA are not likely to be perceived as threatening in themselves. However, the residents are asked to evaluate staff behaviors and institutional policy, and even if the evaluation is only in terms of who makes the decisions, rather than the quality of the decisions made, continued reassurance as to the confidentiality of the data is important. A statement that such data were not shared with the caregivers or the administrators in the settings would be reassuring to the reader.

The other subjects are not likely to find the instruments threatening, although assurance as to confidentiality and anonymity is important here to the nursing assistants. Because interview is not mentioned for this set, the inference is that they completed the instruments privately and in anonymity.

3. *Were the instruments developed by the investigator, or freely adapted from other instruments?* The Resident Questionnaire (RQ) and the Measure of Environmental Support for Autonomy (ESA) were developed by the investigator, and developmental information is not given for these tools. Some reliability information is provided for the SCDA, although the population in which the SCDA was tested is not described.

4. *For original or adapted instruments, how were they developed?* The decision as to what information would be collected and how it would be categorized and described is not discussed. To the extent that the items are described in the results section, it is clear that the items reflect the study concepts. The framework is pragmatic; the intent is to seek information about the three aspects of the environment of interest to the investigator, and the items appear to provide that information.

5. *What tests for reliability and validity were made?* The necessary information is provided for the SCDA, although it is not clear in what population the instruments were tested. Reliability and validity data for the investigator-made instruments are not given. However, the RQ and the ESA, as described, are ostensive and descriptive; content validity is obvious in the items, and neither reliability nor other forms of validity need further consideration. In this exploratory phase of a larger study (p. 364), the lack of such data does not taint the findings, which are mainly straightforward analyses of the frequency of the responses.

6. *How are the instruments scored?* The scoring techniques for the SCDA are reported clearly and comprehensively in the

results section of the article (p. 366). The reader is fully informed as to the source of the numbers in the tables, and the inferences made from the scores as to perception of control are plausible. The information about the scoring formats would have been useful when the instruments were discussed, but it was not hard to find and is also useful where it is. There is less information about the scoring format for the investigator-developed instruments. Judging from the items reported (pp. 365, 367, 368), these data are categorical, consisting of forced choices from a yes-no-uncertain set. Again, scoring is straightforward, and data are presented in terms of how many subjects assigned themselves to each category.

7. *Do the instruments provide the information necessary to test all the research hypotheses or to answer all the research questions?* The instruments provide data to allow the purpose of the study to be met. Characteristics of the three aspects of the environment related to the autonomy of the residents are delineated by means of the perceptions of the inhabitants of the environment.

Application of Instruments to Subjects

1. *What does the investigator do to the subjects, or what must the subjects do, to provide the information necessary to test the hypothesis?* Subjects must submit to a semistructured interview (the residents) or complete a questionnaire (the personnel). The interview is not described in terms of where it occurred or how long it took. The data collection from personnel is also not described, and the fact that it is questionnaire completion and not interview is simply a reasonable assumption by the reader.

2. *In experimental design, how was the independent variable manipulated?* This question is not applicable to this exploratory study.

3. *How were extraneous variables controlled?* This question is not applicable to this exploratory study. The collection of demographic information from the staff and the residents reflects some effort to identify possibly extraneous variables and allows the description of the characteristics of the subjects.

4. *Will the manipulation and control procedures test the hypotheses?* This question is not applicable to this exploratory study.

5. *What are the likely sources of bias in the data-collection techniques?* The author does not provide enough information to make this assessment. The number of interviewers is not given, nor is the time frame for the study. If there were several interviewers over a short period, the question of interviewer training should be considered. If there was only one interviewer, the investigator, over a long period, questions of interviewer fatigue, interviewer training, and possibly systematic bias should be considered. The average length of time and the place of interview

are not noted, so that questions of subject fatigue and privacy are not answered. A set of institutionalized subjects with a mean age of 80.93 years may need a comfortable and private place to respond and a fairly short interview time.

The response directions to the personnel subjects are not given; it is not clear whether they completed instruments at home or on duty, as individuals or as a group. A better description of the data-collection activities would provide information about these and other possible sources of bias.

RESULTS

1. *Does the analysis deal with all of the information obtained that is relevant to the questions asked or the hypotheses tested?* Because the instruments are not fully described, it is not possible to know if all the information is presented. However, in an exploratory design, which data to report lies more with the discretion of the investigator than is possible in experimental design, since the object of exploration is to obtain insights and to identify variables that may or may not be used in a more rigorous study. This investigator analyzes and discusses those data that are useful to the intent to delineate characteristics of three aspects of the environment. The delineation is mainly through the perceptions of the people who inhabit the environment, as these are reflected in the answers to the questions.

2. *Does the investigator present the rationale for a particular analysis?* No, but in this study this is not necessary. The statistical manipulations (percentages, means, and standard deviations) are straightforward and grow out of the characteristics of the data collected.

3. *Do the findings test the hypotheses and/or answer the research questions?* The findings allow the purpose of the study to be met.

4. *Are the categories of response developed correctly?* Information is not presented about the development of categories as such, but the scoring techniques described in the results section suggest that the categories are set up according to the research purpose and meet the rest of the requirements for the development of categories.

5. *Are the statistical manipulations descriptive or inferential?* They are descriptive. The investigator does not generalize the findings to specified populations.

INTERPRETATIONS AND IMPLICATIONS

1. *Are all of the inferences firmly based in the findings?* Yes. The author uses the findings to raise questions about staff edu-

cation, staff perception of residents as impaired and in need of help, the medical model in nursing homes, and methods of implementing inexpensive strategies to develop resident autonomy. This is in no way a misuse, since the findings as reported lend themselves to these questions.

2. *Are the interpretations lodged in the literature?* Yes. In the excellent discussion section, the author uses findings by other investigators to explain and give significance to the findings in the current study.

3. *Does the investigator address the implications of her interpretations?* Yes. Implications of the findings for nursing practice and for nurses' behavior are addressed in the discussion, and the final four paragraphs in the discussion section tie together the study findings, the literature, and the implications of the two for service and research.

In summary, this article is a good example of an exploratory design, which was apparently developed as the initial portion of a larger design addressing relationships between control and morale. As is proper in exploratory work, the conclusions are tentative. However, the study findings are suggestive for that body of nursing knowledge concerned with decision making in the health-care setting.

In the absence of information about the larger study, the report of the exploratory design, the findings it generated, and the analysis and interpretation of those findings must stand alone.

This reader of research is hampered by the absence of research questions identifying the variables and relationships of interest to the author. It is clear from the abstract that data were collected from several groups, and the groups were compared on the variable of perception of self-determination of residents, actual, and the variable of preferred self-determination of residents. These comparative data were used to describe the aspects of the environment of interest to the author. The movement from the purpose of the study to the variables that allow the purpose to be met could have been and should have been described by the author in explicit terms, and this probably was done in the larger study.

The problem could be formulated from the literature, and a major strength of this study is in the logical progression from the background section to the purpose, the methodology, and the interpretation of the results in light of the literature, and the problem.

The sample selection technique was clear and protection of human subjects clearly in place for one set of subjects, the residents. Similar information should have been provided for the rest of the subjects, since status coercion may have been an issue for the nursing personnel (the director said I have to fill out this questionnaire, so I had better do it) and anonymity is always an issue when there is a targeted sample of small size (the administrators).

More information about the instruments would be useful, including the number of questions, the length of time it takes to administer either the interview or the questionnaires, where the data were collected, and by whom. Reliability and validity information is less important for reports of exploratory work, but it is always useful to know how the items were selected and developed. The description of the scoring techniques is comprehensive and clear, although it comes a little late in the article.

There is not enough information provided about the data-collection technique for the reader to identify likely sources of bias, and these are not addressed by the author.

The results section is excellent. The author develops her findings around the aspects of the environment noted in the purpose. Both the tables and the narrative explication are clear, and the author does not combine presentation of the findings with interpretation of the findings, so that it is always obvious to the reader when she is presenting what she found and when she is saying what it might mean.

The tables provide all the necessary information: the percentage tables include the N, and the table of means also provides standard deviations and Ns. The statistics are appropriate to the study.

The discussion section pulls the study components together: the results are lodged in the literature and the implications for nursing are identified. Although the study is described as exploratory by the investigator, who does not generalize the findings, practicing nurses may find some interesting suggestions for alterations in care behavior in the data reported. At the least, the findings are useful as consciousness-raising factors. However, it should be noted that implicit in the discussion is an understanding, possibly based in the morale studies (p. 363), that decision making by patients is a good thing in itself, and nurses *should* be persuaded to support it.

INDEX